Yoga

for Weight Loss

Yoga

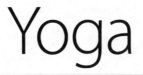

for Weight Loss

Loren Fishman, MD

WITH

Carol Ardman

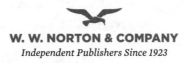

W. W. NORTON & COMPANY

Independent Publishers Since 1923

Yoga for Weight Loss is a general information resource and not a substitute for medical care. Check with your healthcare professional before embarking on any new exercise or weight-loss program. Some yoga poses are contraindicated for certain medical conditions; please read the noted contraindications and do not attempt poses that are not appropriate for you; seek professional advice if you are unsure whether or not to proceed. Follow the instructions for each pose carefully. Even stretching can cause injuries if it's done incorrectly, and poses that are offered as substitutes for the principal poses, to make the poses easier for the beginner, may in some cases carry more risk of injury.

For information about permission to reproduce selections from this book, write to Permissions, W. W. Norton & Company, Inc., 500 Fifth Avenue, New York, NY 10110

For information about special discounts for bulk purchases, please contact W. W. Norton Special Sales at specialsales@wwnorton.com or 800-233-4830

Manufacturing by Lake Book Manufacturing
Book design by Molly Heron
Production manager: Lauren Abbate

ISBN: 978-0-393-35490-4 (pbk.)

W. W. Norton & Company, Inc., 500 Fifth Avenue, New York, N.Y. 10110
www.wwnorton.com

W. W. Norton & Company Ltd., 15 Carlisle Street, London W1D 3BS

1 2 3 4 5 6 7 8 9 0

TO THOSE WHO GENEROUSLY
SHARED THEIR SUCCESS STORIES WITH US,
AND TO ALL THOSE WHO DECIDE TO USE YOGA
AS A TOOL TO CREATE A HEALTHIER FUTURE

Contents

Yoga
for Weight Loss

The Yogic Approach

THINKING ABOUT LOSING WEIGHT—do I need to do it, can I do it, how to do it—can be worrying, even scary. At least that's how it has been for many among my family and friends. One way to figure out how to lose weight is to break the process down into small, meaningful segments. Then these small chunks can be tackled one at a time. Like the Romans of old, we can "divide and conquer." Yoga is particularly adaptable to this approach.

That's what I aim to do in this book, which is for people at any level of experience. What the beginner needs is an overall concept of yoga, and this can also happily remind the experienced practitioner. What follows is mostly about yoga poses, or asana, but does not begin or end there. If you were or are undecided about whether you need to lose weight, here are some things to think about that may help you make a decision and, if necessary, a change in your attitude or your lifestyle.

In spite of persuasive evidence that overweight is inadvisable from medical, social, economic, and aesthetic points of view, the people in many countries are getting rounder. Millions upon millions don't seem to care about the negative consequences. The question is, Why? If we understand why so many people are not moved by the facts, we may get an idea of how to help.

When I tried to understand from the evidence how all these different factors did not deter more people from overeating, I found two powerful currents uniting into a mighty stream. One is evolutionary: the urge to eat.

The motivation to find something edible is an extremely deep and critical one. Obviously, without it few creatures have a chance to survive, let alone procreate. The other explanation is social: Eating is often a social or even recreational activity. And on top of that, growing, baking, marketing, and selling food are obvious ways to offer something people want. Reasonable creatures that we usually are, we look for ways to produce things that our fellow beings want, in order to give our work value, be it on the farm, in the home, or at the market.

So it seems to me that these two conditions, one promoting the survival of the creatures with strong appetites, and the other prompting us to supply the food these creatures really like, have resulted in an almost irresistible coupling of the motivation to eat what is available, with a tremendous worldwide industry to make available the most tempting foods possible. No wonder that our waistlines have grown in tandem with our control over nature—from irrigation to gene modification. We humans have learned over the centuries to supply ourselves with almost irresistible satisfactions for the desires that have developed and amplified in us over millions of years. But then how does one acquire any mastery over this desire, which gives us both the motivation and the means to be so unhealthily, unsocially, uneconomically, and unaesthetically satisfied?

History gives us examples of humankind resisting strong, evolutionarily honed impulses: Social opprobrium and the law stop us from acting out the inappropriate ideas or fantasies put in our heads by very attractive clothing on people of our desired gender. In this case we use willpower or fear of the consequences. These methods of curtailing natural desires have, however, failed quite spectacularly in the case of eating. Conventional means of curbing this desire—outlawing large sugary soft drinks, raising consciousness about fried food, reasoning about diabetes—are too feeble to win against the strength of human appetite. What types of motivation might work?

The abstract ones. People will even die for their ideals. Religious teaching and political mandate have made the very strongest urges, the sexual ones, go into prolonged suspended animation. Yoga is not religion, but yoga can awaken the spiritual impulse, possibly a sentiment strong enough to counter the desire to eat more than one should.

Yoga is theistic, but it has no clergy, no hierarchy, and no churches, temples, or mosques. It has been said that yoga concerns the essence common to all religions. At any rate, the spiritual impulse is alive and thriving in so many yoga practitioners—atheistic and orthodox alike—that it can hardly be a coincidence. Sensing the sanctity of the world, and especially of one's own body, is key to the success of yoga in weight loss. The reader will encounter a detailed discussion of this below. But that is not all yoga offers.

Yoga also offers methods to straightforwardly use your own physiology to reduce your appetite and govern your other functions such as metabolism and sleep, which gives you a veridical sense of mastery over yourself. As the noted philosopher Ludwig Wittgenstein remarked, "The human body is the best picture of the human soul." Effective bodily control is a potent inducement to both self-discipline and a deservedly increased belief in your own self-worth.

Practicing yoga yields a familiarity with yourself—a working knowledge of your own body—that is not easily obtained elsewhere. First, yoga has been shown in innumerable studies to lower anxiety and the effects of stress, which, for many, naturally lead to overeating.[1] If you get to know your own body through yoga, you learn how to regulate stress and its beneficial as well as harmful consequences. In this book I delve into both well-known and rather esoteric physiological ways that yoga cuts down your actual physical appetite and boosts your metabolism. Before this writing, some of this information hasn't, so far as I know, been related directly to yoga.

This makes three basic ways in which yoga holds promise for those who would like to or need to weigh less:

1. Ways to improve your respect for yourself and your world
2. Specific physiological ways to reduce your appetite
3. Systemic ways to improve your metabolism—the process your body uses when it changes the food you've eaten into energy or stores it as fat

Positive outcomes like the ones you'll find described throughout this book occur when all three of these methods combine synergistically.

CHAPTER 1

Tangible and Intangible Yoga Influences

YOGA MAY BE the most effective and innocuous means of limiting or reducing your weight. It not only curtails your appetite in significant ways and improves your ability to generate energy from what you do eat, it also raises your self-esteem, boosts your confidence that you can do what needs to be done, and, possibly most important of all, gives you a sense of the sanctity of your own life, both physical and nonphysical. It is this almost moral, possibly spiritual feature of yoga practice that can infuse you with the motivation needed to overcome so formidable an adversary as the intense, sometimes irresistible, desire to eat.

But what you want to know—the most pressing question to answer—is: How, in practical terms, does yoga help you lose weight? There are six reasons to do yoga if you want to be slimmer.

1. It regulates your appetite. Apart from the physiological effects of yoga on your appetite center, daily yoga also changes your bodily self-perception. You are more mobile, flexible, and ready to act. Many people will feel lighter. After feeling that way a couple of times, and liking it, then comparing it with the feeling after a heavy meal, you learn that

there are pleasures other than the culinary, and that eating differently means feeling better. It's like a very long-lasting mood.

2. It changes what you eat. The lifestyle-change advocates of the last thirty years—Nathan Pritikin, Dean Ornish, and Andrew Weil, to name just three—recommend less fried food, less sugar, less processed food, and more vegetables. Books like *Forks over Knives*, a best-seller with recipes, by Gene Stone, and *The Acid Watcher Diet*, by Dr. Jonathan Aviv, do the same. Yoga's subtle effects encourage the exact same behavior advocated by these experts, who are considered gurus. Yogis eat lots and lots of vegetables.

    New work is beginning to confirm that a number of edible plants promote PGC-1alpha production (more about that fascinating substance, along with mitochondria and telomeres, later), and confer protection on antidiabetic pathways. In addition, nonbarbecued foods and bright-colored fruits and vegetables appear to be larger parts of the diets of people with longer telomeres and longer, fuller lives.

3. It increases your general metabolism by raising the number and activity level of the mitochondria. The exact calculation of how many extra calories you'll burn has never been made, but the good silhouettes, fitness, and high functioning of a majority of serious yogis attest to the virtues of PGC-1alpha, the in-body stimulus for more and more-productive mitochondria. That means converting more glucose into energy, instead of accumulating it as fat.

4. It supports you. Through a combination of diet and the help of support groups, Weight Watchers has built a benevolent empire. Years ago it changed from being a diet company to using group meetings to promote a line of low-calorie foods, a point-system to measure the effect of those foods, and a lifestyle that was new to their clients. The peer-group element as a means of affirming that lifestyle appears to be one of the open secrets about the company's subsequent success. Those people who go to yoga classes have a built-in peer group that actually lives in a healthful way across the board. While the members of the group may or may not change, while no one is weighed once a week, the group dynamic is somewhat similar to that of Weight Watchers. The differences include the previous absence of products,

benefits for the whole body and soul, not just for the numbers on the scale, and very low or no cost.

5. Self-discipline would seem to be the essence of weight control, and yoga promotes self-control like little else. In a sense, self-discipline is just the art of listening to yourself. When you resolve to do something, it is self-discipline that has you following your own imperative. The concept gets elevated to a virtue when your resolve is contrary to your desires. Then it takes some inner strength to stick to your plans. Yoga can help you develop that type of follow-through on your intentions. People are sometimes amazed to find they are actually doing yoga daily. "I've never been consistent with anything like this before" is a comment I've heard more than once. As in a Honda advertisement years ago, yoga "sells itself," invoking a virtuous cycle without extraneous intervention.

6. A positive attitude that is almost a corollary of self-discipline, an inner "Yes I can," is prompted and continued by the observation that you are faithfully doing the yoga. What is willpower if not a combination of positive attitude and powerful self-discipline?[1]

There are many less-tangible but important reasons that yoga helps with weight management. According to what we currently know, yoga began as a program for self-advancement, for liberation from the uncertainties and perceived meaninglessness of this world. However, the elegant beauty and simple relaxation of its practice have led both Western and Eastern minds in the opposite direction—right back to the practical realities of our lives. Like an ethereal pendulum, vital interest in yoga has swung from the rare realms of eternal peace and Nirvana to day-to-day matters of pragmatic concern. The past twenty years have seen an exuberant focus on applying yoga to problems right here on Earth. It has been scientifically proven to help with medical issues such as back pain, post-traumatic stress disorder, cancer, high blood pressure, and many others. And while not proven, it can help, I believe, with world peace.

Ancient yogis lived in various ways. Some did yoga while leading an otherwise normal life, as do most contemporary yoga enthusiasts, who have children, jobs, and many interests and activities. Others lived in groups, often in wild surroundings, self-consciously isolated from society; still others were attached to the great houses of the wealthy, serving as spiritual guides, tutors for the children, and physicians. Two of these three functions are still in evidence, with meditation and mindfulness leading the spiritual way, and many clinicians adopting yoga to solve practical medical problems ranging from the comorbidities of cancer chemotherapy to age-old concerns such as insomnia and overweight.

Spirituality is implicit in the practice, the way beauty in some Japanese drawings is in the spaces between the lines. These "higher" effects will help in the practical application of yoga to the sometimes simple, sometimes complex endeavor of losing weight.

This is possible. Believe it. To bolster your confidence in using this ancient method for this current enterprise, it may be helpful to review the already-proven medical benefits of yoga. Many of these medical conditions that yoga can help treat or cure are associated with overweight. And throughout this book, I will give you advice for how to do yoga poses if you are overweight and have a medical condition frequently associated with it.

CHAPTER 2

Benefits for Conditions Related to Overweight

MEDICAL

HYPERTENSION (HIGH BLOOD PRESSURE)

One of the most startling and, at the same time, most intuitively reasonable discoveries about yoga was Herbert Benson's "relaxation response." Yoga-based meditation was found to reliably reduce high blood pressure by ten to twenty points. Dr. Benson, a Harvard psychiatrist, published his early research more than forty years ago to a skeptical medical establishment, but over the next decades his results have been replicated, prescribed, and utilized many times.[1]

DIABETES

Dr. Kim Innes and some other investigators in India have documented positive changes or remedy for type 2 diabetes with a combination of yoga and dietary wisdom, often also combining meditation and physical postures.[2]

CORONARY ARTERIAL DISEASE

Numerous studies have confirmed that a combination of yoga and lifestyle changes (often brought about by doing yoga) significantly widen the working diameters of the coronary arteries, freeing up blood flow. A number of prominent researchers continue to refine dietary and exercise protocols, mostly centering on the lifestyle changes promoted by yoga practice.[3]

ASTHMA

Since Pranayama and other breathing exercises have long been a staple of yoga, asthma was an obvious application. The great yoga teacher B.K.S. Iyengar is said to have begun yoga as a child because of pulmonary difficulties. The evidence for using yoga to relieve asthma is still somewhat controversial, but a fair number of studies document improved respiration among asthma patients doing yoga.[4]

STRESS

Working at the same Harvard lab in which Walter B. Cannon in the 1920s had discovered the famous "fight or flight" reaction to perceived danger, Herbert Benson, MD, the professor of psychiatry, found the "rest and digest" response to meditation. As perceived danger elevates the heart rate and prepares one for hasty retreat or battle, meditation induces calm and lowers psychological pressure. Benson's results have been replicated many times, even in adolescents without any evidence of hypertension.[5]

LOWER BACK PAIN

Lower back pain is the biggest medical reason for beginning the practice of yoga. The many causes of lower back pain must be identified and treated individually, but once the cause of someone's back pain is properly diagnosed, yoga can provide immediate and long-term benefit. Even treating just the symptoms of back pain or sciatica has proved successful. When studies are done on specific conditions, such as herniated lumbar disc or spinal stenosis, the positive results are likely to be even more dramatic. In general, yoga is clearly effective.[6]

CANCER

No one has yet claimed that yoga cures cancer, but many notable studies affirm that yoga is of substantial aid after surgery and radiation, and during and after chemotherapy. The benefits include not only better range of motion, strength, and posture but also improved mental status, better socialization, and less depression.[7]

OSTEOPOROSIS

A twelve-minute yoga protocol I developed during fifteen years of clinical research has been shown to build bone in people with osteopenia and osteoporosis, as well as in normal individuals who do not want either condition. Advanced age does not seem to interfere with yoga's effective improvement of bone mineral density.[8]

ARTHRITIS

Many different joints may be involved in arthritis, and arthritis takes many different forms, but if yoga does anything, it stretches your muscles, increasing the end points of movement that are almost invariably compromised by arthritis. Here, again, the jury is still out, but many publications confirm the benefits of yoga for arthritis, including rheumatoid arthritis.[9]

DEPRESSION

Strong results from a number of different studies using quite disparate forms of yoga, from Tantric meditation to a standard hatha yoga headstand, have given rise to many yoga-based treatments for depression.[10] Yoga seems to alter your current mood, but it does not necessarily stop there: It can lift your entire "take" on life.

SCOLIOSIS

Since the virtual eradication of polio, and reduced incidence of cerebral palsy, more than 90 percent of scoliosis arises in teenage and preteen girls. We physicians disguise our ignorance of its cause(s) by calling it "idiopathic." Both adolescent idiopathic scoliosis and the degenerative scoliosis that occurs later in life respond well to one or two simple yoga poses, as is shown in radiological before-and-after studies.[11]

ROTATOR CUFF SYNDROME

A single yoga maneuver has been shown to relieve both shoulder pain and the loss of range of arm movement that comes with rotator cuff syndrome.[12]

That maneuver is now being used in a National Institutes of Health (NIH) study on pain.[13]

ANXIETY
A wide variety of yogic techniques have demonstrated efficacy in lowering anxiety on the standard tests measuring anxiety.[14] As in depression, changes can be seen both immediately, while actually doing yoga, and in the longer term, after doing yoga.

POST-TRAUMATIC STRESS DISORDER (PTSD)
Through its calming "parallel play," yoga is often stunningly effective with these warriors wounded more deeply than a surgeon's knife could ever reach. More than 125 Veterans Administration hospitals and clinics have responded to the positive research by using yoga to treat PTSD.[15]

YOGA HELPS IN OTHER WAYS, REGARDLESS OF WEIGHT

So far we have reviewed the strictly medical applications of yoga; they are more or less treatments for diseases that people have. But what about the people themselves? Yoga can work its magic on the normal faculties of people who do not suffer from any disease. This is crucial, because while overweight may be epidemic, while it may cause various medical conditions, overweight itself is not a disease.

MEMORY
Yoga's capacity to improve your short-term and medium-term memory has been demonstrated in numerous studies and almost innumerable anecdotes. Part of its effect relates to practitioners' being calm enough to pay more attention, and part of it appears to be an actual increase in their cognitive capacity.[16]

POSTURE
Due to its focus on the spine, one of the earliest effects of yoga on new students is a beneficial change of carriage. This carries over into better breathing, less back pain, fewer falls, and better self-image and confidence.[17]

BALANCE

Balance is a complex phenomenon. First there is the noun that refers to the equilibrium that disappears when you lose your balance. This type of balance can be a static thing, and its loss can occur while you are simply standing. Then there is the art and skill of balanc*ing*—the verb—a skill people demonstrate in gymnastics and most other sports and also in attempting to regain their balance. Both in the sense of sustaining vertical equilibrium and in the sense of gracefully executing various movements, yoga has been shown to help significantly.[18]

STRENGTH AND RANGE OF MOTION

Through its sustained and extreme positioning, yoga contributes to both your strength and your flexibility.[19] As you age, these assets become increasingly important for your physical and mental well-being.

EXECUTIVE FUNCTION

Sophisticated studies validate the claim that yoga improves healthy people's ability to perform a large variety of simple and complex tasks after they have had a medical issue such as a stroke.[20]

PREGNANCY

Much evidence verifies prenatal yoga as a way to ease the birthing process.[21]

GENERAL COORDINATION

A high-tech electrophysiological study of children in India confirms that enhanced performance is possible after as little as eight weeks of yoga.[22] This includes hand-eye coordination.

THICKENED CORTICAL LAYER FIVE IN THE BRAIN

Of the six layers of cells in our cerebral cortices, yoga's greatest influence appears to be in layer five. Each layer has a large variety of functions, but it is known that thinning is associated with mental decline. In a study done on older people, whose cortices were thinning, yoga appeared to restrain and reduce that degenerative process.[23]

SELF-ESTEEM

Neuropsychological testing reveals the improved self-image and confidence obtained from even eight weekly yoga sessions.[24] In a world rocked by overdose and self-undervaluation, this may be one of yoga's greatest gifts.

WEIGHT LOSS

Though this whole book is about yoga and weight loss, I include weight loss in this long list of yoga's benefits. It's sometimes been a little controversial, but in my experience it belongs here with yoga's amazing benefits. I firmly believe yoga can go a long way toward helping with weight control, and it can do it in a number of ways.[25]

CHAPTER 3

Do You Really Need
to Lose Weight?

BY NOW YOU MAY BE convinced that yoga is powerful enough to help you get slimmer. But the question may arise, as it does for so many procrastinations and avoidances in life: Is this really necessary? Isn't the world full of different opinions of what the "right" weight is? Is there a truly proper weight, anyway? Maybe it's like dresses or suits: One size doesn't fit all, and there are many different situations, and many different styles and tastes, all acceptable.

"One size fits all" *does not* fit the human body. An early attempt to recognize this was the somatotyping system of William Herbert Sheldon, a psychologist in the 1940s. He identified three categories of human body types:

1. Ectomorph (thin, delicate, rapid metabolism, trouble gaining weight)
2. Mesomorph (large boned and well muscled, hard, athletic, "rectangular shape")
3. Endomorph (round shape, fatty tissue, slow metabolism, trouble losing weight)

The names were derived from the three fundamental tissues found in the developing embryo: *ectoderm* (skin and nervous system), *mesoderm* (muscle and bone), and *endoderm* (digestive system). Sheldon even tried to define people's emotional and temperamental types with this system, but that really didn't work. Worse yet, some people seemed to change from one type to another, such as around Christmastime. In the final analysis, the system did not prove definitive.

In 1998, the United States adopted a more quantitative scale, the body mass index, or BMI, invented by Lambert Adolphe Jacques Quetelet, a Belgian mathematician who had applied mathematical methods to the life sciences in the early nineteenth century. The reasoning was that people do not grow like weeds, adding weight directly according to their height (a linear measure), and they do not add weight like pumpkins, through greater spherical radii, which would involve the third power, or cube, of increased size. People grow and develop somewhere in between these models. So Quetelet's index is the weight (in kilograms) divided by the square of the height (in meters).*

The BMI is really a general tool best used for large groups of people. It has to be taken with a grain of salt when applied to individuals, but it does give us definite guidelines: An index value of less than 18 is underweight; normal weight is between 18 and 25; overweight goes from 25 to 29.9; and a person with a BMI above 30 is classified as obese. So if we do the math, if you're 5'4" tall, and weigh 146 pounds, you're overweight. If you weigh 175, you're obese. At 6'1", 190 makes you overweight, and 228 puts you into obesity. You can look at your place on this scale; it is informative.

Now, this system has a few limitations. One equation does not exactly fit all—not both genders, not every age group, not all ethnic groups. Women naturally have fattier skin than men, and that integumentary system is our largest organ. In addition, there are even some ethnic or racial differences in metabolism. These differences are not huge, but they have each been proved by large and accurate studies.

Taking these factors into account, Professor David Fah of Geneva, Switzerland, has helped to introduce the Smart Body Mass Index, or SBMI. I am not impressed with the intelligence of the "smart" BMI. Its cutoff points are far too generous, and it is still quite insensitive to the numerous ways in which one individual differs from another. If a system is going to be smart, shouldn't it consider that hypertension, arthritis, and diabetes have major influences on what your healthy weight should be?

As we age we are advised by the promoters of the Smart Body Mass Index

---

* To calculate yours, use the calculator at the secure website of the National Heart, Lung, and Blood Institute: https://www.nhlbi.nih.gov/health/educational/lose_wt/BMI/bmicalc.htm.

to gain some weight (one suggestion is a pound per year over age sixty) in order to have reserves in case of illness or digestive malfunction. I think that is generally good advice, unless you are obese to start with. Even in concept this system is imperfect, too; while it promotes gaining weight with age to improve survival in serious conditions, it also stresses the nonfat portion of your body: visceral organs, bone, blood, tendon, ligament, nerve, and muscle. Of them, the only one whose mass *we can change* is muscle. Augmenting muscle mass is strongly encouraged in the Smart BMI as adding to the healthy aspect of your weight as you age. However, we know that muscle mass increases energy expenditure, even at rest, which will of course tend to deplete the very energy reserves that the system is trying to protect in older people.

Neither of these systems is perfect, but from all the experience I've had as a physician, the BMI is the best place to start, with modification to people's ideal weight adjusted by their individual conditions.

Unfortunately there appears to be no definitive way for you to decide what measures to use when figuring out just how overweight or unhealthily underweight you are. So I recommend using the BMI, tempered by additional considerations. If you have hypertension or diabetes, lower the number you calculate by 5–7 percent to get a more accurate BMI; if you have a tendency toward anorexia, or a chronic digestive condition, raise the number accordingly. As this is the best we can do at present, I think this is the most practical and beneficial way to take a reading on your current weight.

These are the apparent state-of-the-art medical ways to tell whether you should stay as you are, lose weight, or gain weight as you age and if so, how much. They also give an idea of whether that adjustment of weight is of medical relevance, a potent source of motivation. For sure, these guidelines do not exhaust the medical *reasons* for lowering weight: Coronary and pulmonary conditions, arthritis, and the efficacy of anticancer drugs all have weight-related consequences. These considerations are all waiting in the wings to strengthen your resolve. We will get to that. Now we must examine the other tests that address the critical first question: Do you need to lose weight?

A PERSONAL SCALE

Many times we are so distracted or otherwise occupied that the medical consequences of overweight—bad things that could happen—do not tip the scales in favor of doing something to slim down. In that case more personal criteria may come into play. If you feel uncomfortable, there is no need to send yourself a memo: You know it right away.

The saying "comfortable in one's own skin" is a place to begin. Getting into or out of the shower, does your abdomen tend to pull you forward? Are your thighs so thick that you cannot sit comfortably in your car? Are intimate positions compromised or even prohibited by your size? These are things you will know in your birthday suit.

Are you out of breath with just one flight of stairs? Do you like what you see in the mirror? When you carry things, does your back begin to ache (because your abdomen prevents holding them close)?

And never mind skin. What about clothing? You might feel uncomfortable if your abdomen pulls your shirt apart between the button and the buttonhole, or if your shoes are confining although the bones of your feet haven't changed in fifteen years.

THE YOGA TESTS

Being an activity that cultivates comfort, agility, and balance, yoga can be used to figure out whether something is impairing your balance, agility, or overall fitness, including strength. Let us begin with balance, something increasingly vital to your well-being as you age, and something that is certainly affected by overweight.

BALANCE

Vriksasana
The Tree (a variation)

Benefits and how it works: Requiring a fair amount of balance, this pose both improves a practitioner's balance and detects poor balance in someone who attempts but cannot really do it. This version of the pose is safe for those who would find the classical pose quite challenging, and yet is still rigorous enough to detect deficits in a person's equilibrium.

Contraindications: Do not attempt this pose if you have plantar fasciitis or a sprained ankle or already know your balance is impaired. With plantar fasciitis or sprained ankle, you can stand on the other foot.

THE POSE

1. Brace the side of a chair against a wall so it faces you when you stand with the chair to your right and your back against the wall.
2. Stand with your feet hip-width apart, toes spread out. Press the ball and heel of your left foot firmly into the floor. Tighten the left quadriceps and hamstrings moderately, making the whole thigh firm. Tuck the buttocks in and move the lower pelvis forward, which will mildly extend your hip. These maneuvers should reduce your lumbar curve.
3. Align your pelvis directly above your feet. Lift your right foot and place it on the seat of the chair, toes pointing away from you.
4. Retain a forward-facing pelvis as you carefully, slowly swing the bent right knee and thigh out to the side (ideally at ninety degrees to the left foot).
5. Fix your gaze on a point at eye level, fifteen to twenty feet away.
6. Slowly inhale as you (optionally—see page 65) raise your arms symmetrically, turning the palms inward to meet above your head, biceps as far behind the ears as possible without making your head go forward. In any event, let your lungs fill completely as you do so.
7. Bring your shoulder blades close together behind you, stretch upward from your left ankle through the crown of your head to the tips of your thumbs and fingers. Advance your torso just enough to stand without the wall's support. Stretch skyward.

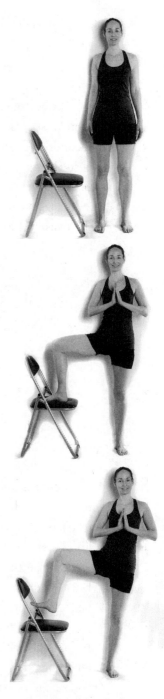

Vriksasana, the Tree

8. Now for the test: Slowly and carefully lift your right foot off the chair. If you start to fall forward, put your foot back down.

9. Now repeat with your left foot on the chair.

If you can hold this position for fifteen seconds, that's great. If you cannot, then balance is something you need to improve. If you can hold it for those few seconds, it doesn't mean you don't need to lose weight, but if you can't hold the pose there's a strong possibility that you need to trim down. Of course, over-weight is not the only cause of imbalance, but if you tend to lose your balance in less than fifteen seconds, you should improve it, even if excess weight is *not* the cause. This is especially important if your performance suggests that your balance is significantly worse than you remember it being in the past. Yoga is just as successful in remediating loss of balance as it is in detecting it.[1] This pose can be advanced as your balance improves. See pages 64–67.

We will go over this pose, and others like it, in significantly greater detail later. At this point it is sufficient to note the results, and move on to whether anything is impairing your ability to move. For this one you go down on the floor.

AGILITY

Marichyasana I
Seated twist (variation)

Benefits and how it works: The ribs keep the thoracic spine from doing much rotation, and the lumbar vertebral facets move forward and back, also restricting any twisting. This leaves only the junction between the thoracic and lumbar spine, T12–L1, to do most of the twisting. However, pressure generated by the twist is sustained throughout the thoracic and lumbar vertebrae. Because of this, the pose is excellent for osteoporosis as well. It is a definite bone builder.

Contraindications: If you have a herniated disc, twist to the opposite side. In facet arthritis or facet syndrome, be gentle with yourself; the other poses recommended here may be better test cases for you. Avoid this pose after abdominal or back surgery and posterior hip replacement.

THE POSE

1. Sit with your legs extended straight out on a rug or soft mat.
2. Press your hands down on the floor beside you to lift your spine.
3. Bend your right knee and place that foot on the mat beside the thickest part of the left thigh.
4. Anchor the left leg firmly down, stretching fully through the sole of the foot. Especially stretch the big-toe side of the foot forward, keeping it vertical.
5. On your next inhalation, lift your spine again and turn toward the right.
6. Place your left upper arm outside your right knee. Slide it forward to engage the outside of the folded knee as high up on the arm as possible without rounding your back. Optionally, raise your forearm and hand to vertical.
7. Press the outside of your knee with the outside of your left upper arm or armpit and slide your left forearm to the left of your right shin, reaching back behind you with the left hand, and walk your right hand back around to the left on the floor for balance. It will also elevate your shoulders and straighten your spine.

Now for the test: Does your abdomen keep you from twisting any further because it is squeezed by the right thigh? Is your left thigh so thick that you cannot twist around it? To examine this, straighten up with each inhalation, and twist a little more as you exhale. Each time you twist, walk your right

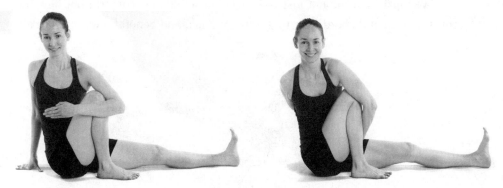

Marichyasana, seated twist

hand around behind you toward the left in order to coax the right shoulder back. Pull your left shoulder blade back to impel your left chest (not the shoulder) forward and to the right. Does buttock flesh give you an unstable balance? Does your left arm fail to slide by your right thigh for lack of space?

A yes to any of these questions means weight and dimension are relevant to your situation. Of course twisting may be difficult because of stiffness, a herniated disc, rotator cuff syndrome, and other factors not related to weight. You can compare your sitting-on-the-floor twist with the same twist standing up with your foot on a chair, as in the first pose above, to see if it is stiffness, or whether the size of your limbs and abdomen is the limiting factor. If you're having trouble judging, get someone to help.

OVERALL FITNESS, INCLUDING STRENGTH AND BALANCE

Kakasana
The Crow

Benefits and how it works: This pose mobilizes almost every part of your body, and therefore affords an excellent opportunity to see how well your body fills your unpredictable needs.

Contraindications: Readers in the second or third trimesters of pregnancy, or with osteoporosis, Dupuytren's contractures, or extreme weakness should avoid this pose.

We must examine not just your balance, agility, or strength, but how the three add up and coordinate to grant you grace and general mobility. We are

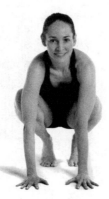
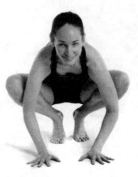
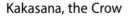

Kakasana, the Crow

not talking about cardiovascular fitness, or suitability for the Navy SEALs, but whether, put bluntly, your muscles match your mass, and together both can achieve a stable, harmonious whole.

In this pose your back is rounded, which can injure those with osteopenia, osteoporosis, herniated lumbar disc, or severe kyphosis, so an alternative pose for those people follows this one.

THE POSE

1. Place a pillow, some folded blankets, or something else soft in the middle of a yoga mat.
2. Stand about one foot behind it.
3. Squat.
4. Place your hands as wide apart as your shoulders. Spread out your thumbs and fingers.
5. Place your knees as high up on your arms as possible.
6. Press your thighs inward into your triceps.
7. Raise your weight up as you come onto the balls of your feet, lifting your heels.
8. Raise your head somewhat, without compressing the back of your neck.
9. Lift first one foot, then the other foot, then both feet off the floor, as you advance more of your weight forward onto your fingers.
10. This is a good position. Hold it, both feet aloft, for at least ten seconds.
11. If you wish to go further, straighten your elbows, transitioning from Kakasana, the Crow, to Bakasana, the Crane.

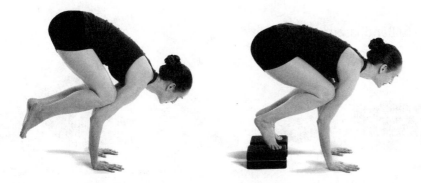

On the other hand, if the Crow seems out of reach, I recommend a simpler way to get into it. Place a block behind you, and after squatting and pressing your thighs against your triceps, lift your feet onto the block, which will raise your weight up and make "liftoff" onto your hands and bent elbows easier.

What stands in the way of accomplishing this pose, which for many can be difficult? Basically it can be weakness in the arms and shoulders, relative to one's weight. It can also be explained by an abdomen so large or thighs so ponderous that they don't fit onto the upper arms. Another more extreme obstacle is so much nonmuscular, nonbone flesh on either the arms or the thighs that one resting on the other is wobbly. Finally, there may be a sense of balance that is overtasked by the total strength-to-weight proportions.

If you happen to have osteopenia, osteoporosis, or a herniated lumbar disc, here is a safe composite measure of how well your strength, weight, and balance match up. The following pose is for the people who couldn't even attempt the Crow because of the contraindications.

Setu Bandhasana
The Bridge

Benefits and how it works: This is an exhilarating posture that quickens heart and mind. It is actually part of the yoga sequence shown to build bone, and is part of many regimens meant to relieve depression.

Contraindications: It should not be done by people with spinal stenosis, anterolisthesis, or facet syndrome. Other contraindications include GERD, herniated cervical disc, severe kyphosis, advanced arthritis, and advanced pregnancy. If any of these conditions applies to you, and you also cannot do the arm balance just described, you might review your past activities with

Setu Bandhasana, the Bridge

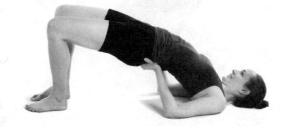

an eye to overall fitness and ask yourself if you're getting out of breath just getting dressed to go out, or if rising from a chair is becoming challenging.

THE POSE

1. Lie on your back with a folded blanket under your shoulders but not under your head. Let your arms remain at your sides.
2. Bend your knees and place your feet squarely on the floor and parallel.
3. Raise your torso off the mat, with the region between your navel and your pubic bone highest. Place your hands, fingers facing toward each other, under your kidney region for support. Elbows should still be at your sides, and forearms vertical.
4. Use your quadriceps and gluteal muscles to put pressure on your feet, as though you were trying to push your feet away from you, but don't actually move your feet. Use the backward force of your legs to generate forward force that will lift your torso and pelvis higher, arching your back, elevating your pubic region, and advancing your chest forward over your throat as much as possible.
5. Retain your arms and hands as before: Support yourself in this higher arch with your hands under your lower back, elbows at right angles, hands pointing toward each other. Remain in the pose for at least thirty seconds. A minute is better.

If this is impossible, if your abdomen just doesn't lift, that is a positive indicator for the need to lose weight and/or get stronger. For a finer appraisal, you might try this easier version:

VARIATION

Strap your elbows together so they are shoulder-distance apart. The strap goes around the arms above the elbows. Lift your pelvis and place your hands underneath your lower back.

If you can do this, but couldn't do the strapless version that precedes it, then the problem is strength, relative to weight, but it is not as serious as being unable to do either version.

In addition to seeing whether you need to lose weight, I have stealthily tried to slip three valuable aids into this self-testing:

1. Raising your confidence that weight change is important, in a personal way, which is bound to heighten your motivation. By now you may agree that weight change can be significant, and if you have, your motivation should be greater.
2. Bolstering confidence in your own abilities to get something done, accomplish something bodily. You have to try: If you have done any of the yoga here, you have accomplished something with your body. I hope that has given you confidence in your own ability.
3. Experiencing it, you may now agree that yoga is not so terrible and impossible as it might once have seemed.

Setu Bandhasana—easier version

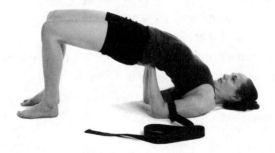

CHAPTER 4

Real People Get Thinner

THE IDEA THAT yoga can help a person lose weight is actually contested by some people, because the rate of metabolism decreases during the practice of many styles of yoga. I believe that claims made by reasonable people that yoga does nothing for weight control are based on misunderstanding and incomplete information. It's true that if your metabolism is working more slowly and converting less food into energy, fewer calories are used. Nevertheless, a number of studies and a large number of individuals bear testimony to yoga's efficacy in long-term weight loss.[1]

This works through biochemical factors, unlike the simple calorie-burning of traditional exercise. Yoga is an effective weight loser even in strict mindfulness training, as we've seen. At the biochemical level, yoga reduces critical hormones such as interleukins and raises hormones such as adiponectin, which goes a long way toward lower inflammation and greater weight loss.

The experience of a fellow I'll call Bryan Wayne is just one of many. He came to me as a patient with back pain about seven years ago. He said it hurt low down on both sides almost every time he moved. Bryan worked for the Parks Department here in New York City and was lifting and moving heavy things like benches and sewer covers for hours every day. He was one of those forty-year-olds you might call "fully packed." If you poked a finger into his abdomen, it bounced back out at you. He was also very stiff in his joints, and it was pretty clear that he didn't do much in the way of deliberate exercise. At 5'9" tall, he weighed 260 pounds.

But he was intelligent, inquisitive, and willing to learn. When I suggested that his stiff joints made him use his back (which was also notably stiff) in ways that were bound to cause pain and injury, he listened. He joined in the conversation, citing examples of how it was true that his surplus weight gave him a lot of extra work and deprived him of many movement options.

"I couldn't lift the bushy trees we were planting last week, because my belly kept me from getting very close to them," he told me. "My knees couldn't bend far enough for me to get under them. There was no way I could lift them up and put them on the cart. So I had to lug them a long way over the grass. That ended up with my back hurting. It hurts right now."

I sent Bryan to Jan, a yoga teacher I work with in my office, for some rudimentary yoga. At first what he was able to do was almost like a pantomime of yoga: hardly any stretching, just a little mobilization. The initial idea was to impress on him that he *could* move and enjoy it. Fortunately, Jan's joy in her student's movement was contagious, and within a few weeks Bryan was not just doing as he was told. He was trying to do better, to imitate what Jan seemed to do so effortlessly and happily. He started trying to do it at home.

Within three months he had lost twenty pounds and 50 percent of his back pain. Then he joined Weight Watchers. After a year or so, seeing Jan once a week, and changing the way he ate, he had lost seventy-five pounds. He found himself doing reasonably skilled yoga, and was pain-free.

Approximately six months later I saw him at a yoga gathering. He was slim, muscular, and had the kind of smile on his face that is hard to manufacture. He saw Jan after that, and now he is thinking of teaching yoga in addition to doing his regular job.

I don't look at Bryan's stint with Weight Watchers as detracting from yoga's influence in his weight loss. Quite the contrary. Weight Watchers had been around for a long time, and what was required for him was enough motivation to *do* something. In a reasonably short time, his not-so-conscious impulses were free enough for him to get serious: to see clearly that he really *could* lose the weight and that this might not be a bad thing.

This man had a realistic but utterly unspiritual sense of his body. Yoga gave him a more liberated way to occupy that body and improved his self-esteem. The yoga itself may not have burned all the calories it took for him to slim down, but it helped him shed the intimidating bodily alienation that keeps so many of the overweight from trying.

Importantly, yoga was also at work on the physiological level. There are a number of positive studies showing that the more you delve into mind-body activities, the less you weigh.[2]

Then there is Stacey Morris. She lost 180 pounds, mostly through yoga, and has kept the weight off for ten years. She had been a chubby kid in a chubby (okay, obese) family, where, she says, she and her father were "eating buddies." Though she began sporadic dieting at the age of nine, it "made her hungrier." The yo-yoing lowered her self-esteem. At one point she weighed more than 300 pounds.

She says, "I was heartbroken in college when a boyfriend started saying about me, 'Oh, you're so disgusting. You've got to change.' I hated myself. You know, a lot of women gain weight to hide from men."

That was one of the things she was doing—hiding in the mountain of her body—while she worked for a decade as a reporter for a daily newspaper. At forty-four she was a freelance writer, focusing on food, travel, and the arts.

The work itself was great, but the unhappy, unhealthy environment exacerbated my stress eating. Being sedentary behind a desk most of the day didn't help either. My plan was to use my writing to become a size-acceptance activist. I even wrote opinion columns to that effect, which was kind of ironic.

In actuality, I was using food as a crutch. I had lost one hundred pounds on a diet in my twenties—in fact I lost and regained one hundred pounds twice. Neither time did it build up my self-esteem or confidence. That had been badly damaged by childhood bullying. So I said, 'Enough. I may be heavy, but that doesn't make me a bad person.' I said to myself, 'I'm going to fix what's inside; what's outside is beyond me.'

Then three things happened: I saw Carnie Wilson, the daughter of Brian Wilson of the Beach Boys, on TV talking about her struggles with weight. Shortly after that I met and got to know the pro wrestler

Diamond Dallas Page, whose weight-loss success with an Ashtanga-based yoga program inspired me. That was just about the time my weight peaked at 345.

I had done Kundalini yoga, but this yoga was new, and I had learned some lessons from my past tries at weight loss. My story is kind of spiritual. Yoga helped me from the inside out. Between carrying the weight and my body being sandbagged by the lousy, processed foods I existed on, I was half-awake a lot of the time compared to now. As I got more into yoga, I gradually woke up, became more aware of myself and everything else, felt much more energetic, found I could do more. Yoga is a great way to de-age your body. I feel and look better now than I did in my twenties.

After I started doing yoga seriously, I broke off an unhappy platonic relationship and was alone for a while. Then I decided to put myself out there, on internet dating sites. The right man came into my life, and now we're engaged to be married.

I stopped eating gluten and cow-dairy products. As I did the yoga, the weight came off without a struggle. The first month of doing lots of yoga I lost twenty pounds! Then it was about ten pounds a month, without it bothering me, making me feel hungry, making me feel deprived. I felt better all the time. Everything in my life came together as the pounds went away. Now I write books, do yoga, and lecture all over the country.

Then there is Jesse Ruggiere, who needed a cardiac ablation and had arthritis and bad knees at the age of thirty. Possibly because of a rare condition called Castleman disease, he developed thyroid cancer and needed to have his thyroid removed. He existed on fast food, soda, and a bottle of Jack Daniels a day. At 5'8" tall he weighed 236 pounds. Jesse's doctor didn't just prescribe exercise—he said Jessie absolutely *had* to exercise.

Watching a YouTube video about DDP (Diamond Dallas Page) Yoga, he thought, If those guys can do it, so can I. Six years later, Jesse weighs 184. He has an abdominal six-pack instead of a six-pack of beer. I asked him if he thinks his yoga has a spiritual aspect. "Everyone has a different definition of spiritual," he said. "What I do is pure workout." But he also says yoga has given him a "totally new life." In that new life, in addition to yoga, Jesse runs the Tough Mudder military race for charity and works out daily. He teaches foster kids that they can be active and move, and he took a group of them to a baseball game—their first. If those activities don't have a spiritual component, I don't know what activities do. His attitude is also one of hope. "Every day is Day One of a health journey."

––––––––––

Neither Bryan, Stacey, Jesse, nor any of the others who were generous enough to share their stories with me in these pages was alone. I admire them for their commitment, for keeping at it, for forging ahead physically, emotionally, and spiritually. They are an inspiration for all those who are overweight. If you are one of those people, it's important to know you belong in a huge group of people like yourself. Here are some mind-blowing facts about overweight that these brave people who embraced yoga didn't know when they began learning both the physical and spiritual aspects of this practice.

OVERWEIGHT IS UBIQUITOUS

No matter what your situation, or whether you consider your need to control your weight mild or extreme, you certainly aren't alone.

According to the United States National Health and Nutrition Examination Survey, 2009–10:[3]

- More than two in three adults are overweight or obese.
- More than one in three adults is obese.
- More than one in twenty adults has extreme obesity.
- About one in three children and adolescents, age six to nineteen, is overweight or obese.
- Half of these children and adolescents are obese.

There are no accurate statistics on just how many yogis are overweight, obese, or morbidly obese, but, assuming you have some familiarity with yoga, as most do, my question is: Have you ever seen a class of yogis two-thirds of whom are overweight? I don't think so. Though there are "big" yogis, both men and women, and they aren't rare, they are very far from being in the majority. The majority are in the "normal" range.

According to the bar graph, in the study years 2009–10, approximately 74 percent of American men were overweight or obese; 64 percent of women were identified with overweight or obesity. Equal percentages (36 percent) of men and women were obese, which means more men than women were just plain overweight. Among men, 4 percent had extreme obesity; the percentage among women was double that of men, at 8 percent.

Roughly speaking, from the 1960s to today, America has gone from being a country in which one-third of the population was overweight or obese to one where more than two-thirds of us are in these categories.[4]

Here is an amazing thought. More than 37 million people are currently doing yoga of some kind.[5] If yoga can actually help people shed pounds, and I believe it can, then if enough people do yoga, it may eventually cause a truly widespread and significant reversal of the nation's unhealthy trend toward obesity.

Estimated Percentage by Sex

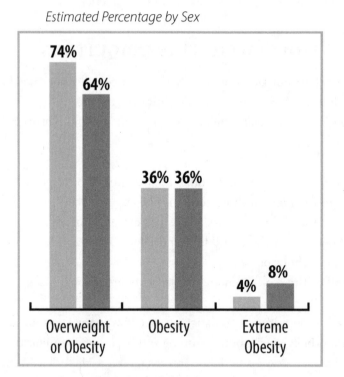

Men are the lighter of the two grays
Women are the darker of the two
Source: NIDDK, "Overweight & Obesity Statistics."

CHAPTER 5

How Yoga Works Deep
Inside Your Body

WE HAVE NOW reviewed some of the trenchant arguments for doing yoga. American yoga has grown from 20.4 million practitioners in 2012 to 36.7 million in 2016. Over 100 million Americans have tried yoga at home. There are more Americans doing yoga than there are in some prominent Christian denominations.[1]

Yes, yoga is that popular. Yet, of course, there are an even larger number of people who have not tried it. *Yoga Journal* and Yoga Alliance have teamed up with Ipsos Public Affairs to find out why some people—some of whom could certainly benefit from its weight-loss properties—shy away from yoga.[2] Here are the five main reasons, along with rejoinders that hopefully will help persuade the skeptical.

1. "I'm not sure if it is right for me." Answer: There's only one way to find out.
2. "I don't know how to get started." Answer: This book contains advice and encouragement. Keep reading!
3. "I don't exercise." Answer: Yoga is not exactly exercise in the usual sense, though when doing poses you are exercising. Still, this may be the right moment to begin to move and stretch.

4. "I feel out of place in a yoga class." Two answers: There are so many yoga teachers and so many yoga classes that there are very likely at least a few that are right and comfortable for any given individual. Also, the instructions in this book can be carried out at home and done almost entirely on your own.

5. "My body is not right for yoga." Two answers: Yoga practitioners of so many different "body types" exist right now that it's unlikely yours is not among them. Also, yoga harmonizes, coordinates, and unifies you and your body, so even if yours were a "non-yoga body," the practice of yoga would likely transform it and change that.

Unlike most of the current methods of weight loss, yoga is practically free, currently requires no license to practice or teach, and has such beneficial "side effects" as more elegant posture, better balance, greater range of motion, improved strength, finer coordination, lower anxiety, and all the other curative properties we reviewed in chapter 1. It is silent, requires no paraphernalia, and is easy to remember. So how, in detail, does yoga transform you from a person who is bigger than you may want to be to someone in your desired range?

YOUR BRAIN AND STOMACH "TALK" TO EACH OTHER

To evaluate the role of yoga in weight loss, we must recognize that the brain, among its many functions, is also part of the digestive apparatus—a good part of why we eat as we do, act as we do, and therefore weigh what we weigh.[3] The illustration on the facing page shows what the stomach, the organ inside us, looks like; it also indicates where the receptors lie, and a few of their linkages with the brain. In the picture, *CNS* abbreviates "central nervous system."

This linkage I refer to isn't only from the stomach to the brain. It includes the part of the esophagus just north of the stomach, and the first part of the duodenum, the intestinal beginnings past the exit-hatch from the stomach. Stretching the stomach and these parts just a little promotes the secretion of the enzymes that aid in digestion: histamine and gastrin and pepsinogen. It also causes the stomach's muscles to contract. However, with an increased

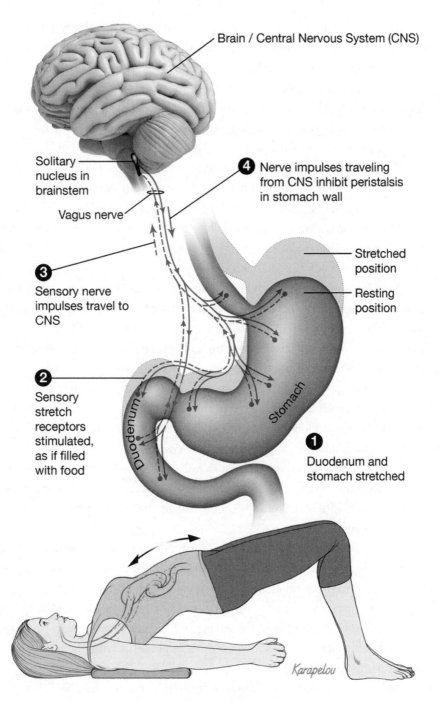

Brain / Central Nervous System (CNS)

Solitary nucleus in brainstem

Vagus nerve

4 Nerve impulses traveling from CNS inhibit peristalsis in stomach wall

Stretched position

Resting position

3 Sensory nerve impulses travel to CNS

2 Sensory stretch receptors stimulated, as if filled with food

Duodenum

Stomach

1 Duodenum and stomach stretched

Karapelou

The flexible digestive system

stretch—more than just a little—the opposite occurs: cholecystokinin and adiponectin hormones emerge. Miraculously, this cuts down the activity of the digestion mechanism and speeds fat metabolism. At the same time the hunger-stimulating hormone ghrelin diminishes sharply, further damping down the desire to eat.[4] Further, and most important, stretching the intestinal, esophageal, and stomach receptors propagates direct feedback to the appetite centers in the brain, inhibiting their function. These stretches rapidly cut down appetite. We immediately become less hungry. Yes, stretching the stomach enough by doing rather simple yoga can actually decrease your desire to eat!

As it turns out, stretching the stomach radially, as if inflating a balloon in the stomach, or eating a large meal, has much more effect on your appetite than stretching this organ the long way—top to bottom.[5] That is exactly what yoga does—stretches the stomach radially.

Focusing down more finely than anatomy, we enter histology, the study of tissues—the aspect of live things that are smaller than organs but larger than cells. These are groups of cells, with their surrounding self-manufactured extracellular elements. Here we can really understand how and why and where and when stretching the tissues of those organs—the lower esophagus, stomach, and upper duodenum—has the greatest effect on appetite.

The duodenum is bound down to the rest of the body at two points, lower down at the hepatoduodenal ligament, where the duodenum gets closest to the liver, and higher up, by the fascia that encompasses the head of the pancreas. See the picture on page 35 for details. When you arch your back, those two points move apart, and the characteristic duodenal arch becomes somewhat flattened. Such stretching is well within the "normal range of motion" of these organs.

Studies have refined the observations made here about the stomach. Let me mention a few of them here to attempt to entice you into learning more about this convenient relationship between stretch and slimness. Actually, a number of animal studies find that stomach stretch is the most important factor in limiting appetite.[6] Some researchers have genetically "removed" this feedback-system loop, which controls appetite in fruit flies. Result: The altered fruit flies are "supersized."

Part A in the illustration shows a fruit fly without a feedback loop from the stomach to the brain. Part B shows a normal fruit fly.

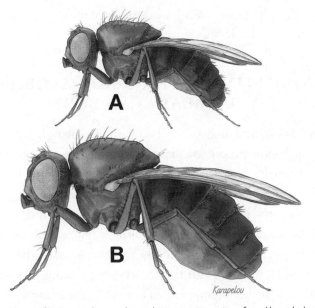

Fruit flies with and without appetite feedback loop

YOUR SENSES AND EMOTIONS
HAVE PHYSICAL EFFECTS

Yet another wonderful and related action takes place when you do yoga. It happens subtly, even without your assent: You are suddenly paying more attention to yourself and everything else. You are more conscious, just plain more aware. This new sensitivity has two aspects: *Interoception* involves those sensations that come from inside you, be it your joints, your sinuses, or your stomach. *Exteroception* involves sensing your environment, including the heat of the day, the sidewalk under your feet, and everything else you feel with your skin, see, hear, smell, and taste. It may not seem obvious, but the yogic heightening of interoceptive acuity is useful for reducing your appetite and losing weight. It supplies another route in addition to the physical stretch, which makes you less hungry.

Many studies confirm that yoga improves interoception, making you more informed of your bodily state and sensations. In other words, the yoga here not only stretches the appetite-curbing receptors but also makes you more keenly responsive to your newly lowered impetus to eat. Yoga becomes a self-enhancing ally in the quest for caloric limitation, a system going in the right direction—toward less food.

NIGHTTIME EATING AND CALORIES YOUR BRAIN CAN BURN

Yoga lowers anxiety, and anxiety can be related to eating long after the regular dinner hour. Some people maintain that eating late at night has a very big effect on your weight. A calorie is a calorie is a calorie, but there is some truth in this: The stretch receptors in the duodenum, stomach, and lower esophagus suppress appetite only one-fourth as powerfully at midnight as they do at noon. So if you go down for a snack in the wee hours of the morning, you'll be likely to eat a substantially greater amount than would satisfy you at lunch. Moreover, the lack of sleep, and the anxiety about facing tomorrow without enough of it, may further prompt you to overeat.[7] Higher anxiety is associated with higher levels of ghrelin, the fat maker, and lower levels of leptin, adiponectin, and the other slimming hormones.[8] You can calm down with yoga.

It is also well documented that your brain is a major calorie burner. I find it amazing that our brains use an estimated 20 percent of the calories we consume, which is another way the brain is linked to the stomach. There are Tibetan yogis who direct their scantily clad acolytes to meditate in the wintry mountain forests, and estimate their proximity to enlightenment by how much snow has melted around them. Yogis may or may not be able to voluntarily stop their hearts, but there is little doubt that they can start their heads, that they can just sit there, apparently motionless, and burn calories.

Actually, yoga styles range from the highly energetic and metabolically demanding regimens of B.K.S. Iyengar and K. Pattabhi Jois to the calmly reflective lagoons of meditation. Some styles of yoga can raise your heart rate, and presumably the rate at which you're turning calories into energy plus carbon dioxide plus water. This, of course, burns calories. Every type and tradition of yoga involves some exercise. Recent science finds that exercise of the yogic kind (as well as other kinds) brings about cellular changes that play right into the plans of those who need and want to control their weight. Contemporary science has solidly proved two such changes, one in the cell, and one within its nucleus.

THE MORE MITOCHONDRIA, THE BETTER FOR WEIGHT LOSS

When it comes to the cell, I am referring to a molecule with the eminently forgettable name of peroxisome proliferator-activated receptor gamma coactivator-1alpha (PGC-1alpha), a fearsome intracellular warrior that reduces arthritis and inflammation of all kinds, and lowers the risk of Alzheimer's disease, heart disease, and a number of cancers. It also accelerates the proliferation of mitochondria, the fat burners of our bodies.[9] Telling you something about the mitochondria here makes sense, since they are almost universally believed to be the strongest ally, in a sense the only ally, of all of us who want to lose weight.[10] And by far the strongest stimulus to create more mitochondria is PGC-1alpha.

Mitochondria originated with a symbiotic relationship between a bacterial and an animal cell. This began when Earth was at least a billion years younger than it is today. The most favored theory is that mitochondria stem from a bacterial cell that was engulfed by an animal cell and for some reason was not digested by the animal cell. Instead, it survived within the animal cell. Before long the bacterial DNA was supplying the animal cell with energy that gave that particular cell a distinct advantage over others. After a while, only these bacterially fortified cells and their progeny survived. The animal cells and the smaller bacterial cells within them had managed to help each other, the bacteria giving the animal cells more energy, and the animal cells protecting their small internal power stations from the great world beyond.

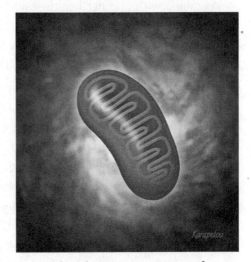

The mitochondria developed over the course of time to supply the cells with almost all their energy, and with that support, the cells specialized into liver, retina, and all the other fabulously coordinated functionality of complex animals and humans. Although both

A mitochondrion, power station of all cells

the cells' nuclei and the mitochondria have DNA, neither could get by, neither could live, without the other. Most of the proteins that mitochondria use come from the cells' nuclei and the DNA in the nuclei. But energy is developed almost solely in the mitochondria, and the structures that produce it come from the mitochondrial DNA. Cells that use more energy have more mitochondria. One liver cell is estimated to have two thousand. Heart muscle may be 40 percent mitochondria. Mitochondria are 10 to 12 percent of our human body weight!

On the molecular level, we really run on electricity. Our hearts contract with the use of electrical impulses, our nerves conduct along very close analogues of electric wires, and our muscles are soft electric motors that ratchet rather than spin. The mitochondria do all the electron transferring. And the more mitochondria there are, the more energy that becomes available for everything we do. Yoga induces your body to release more PGC-1alpha, which induces more mitochondria, which in turn changes more glucose into energy. This makes for a slimmer, more energetic person.

How does PGC-1alpha make for more mitochondria? True to their bacterial origins, mitochondria can glom together and also divide quite independently of the cells that host them. If the DNA or other structures in a single mitochondrion are damaged or degraded, the mitochondrion finds a way to combine with another healthy one to restore their all-important function. If the cell is in need of more energy, there are mechanisms within the cell that prompt the mitochondria to split in two and thus increase their numbers. As is so frequently the case in nature, there are checks and balances. Each cell also generates forces that limit the number and activity of the mitochondria. But the prime factor for increasing their number is PGC-1alpha.

So what does this mean for the person intent on losing weight? More, and more active, mitochondria translate directly into a more energetic, more metabolically active life. The greater the number of mitochondria in your liver, the better it functions, handling glucose production and use, and secreting enzymes to digest fats. More mitochondria in cartilage cells means healthier and better-moving joints that are less susceptible to arthritic degradation. The same goes for stronger and more resilient tendons, a more accurately responsive immune system, a more finely regulated thyroid gland, extra-retentive memory cells, and more-discriminating appetite centers in your brain. It makes for a higher-functioning *you*. When it comes to weight loss, you use additional calories to live better and you become a higher-functioning organism.

Mitochondrial enrichment is about as deep-seated and pervasive a change as anyone can make. Yoga usually slows your metabolism *while you are doing it*, but after practicing it for some time, it raises your energy utilization generally. Saying that yoga cannot help you lose weight because it lowers your metabolism is similar to saying that higher education cannot improve your income because when you're in school you make no money and in fact have to pay for it. On the contrary, yoga enables you to convert calories into a better and finer life for yourself.

Physicians are fond of saying, "As you get older, your metabolism slows down," to account for what has been called middle-age spread. There are many reasons for this change in so many people's bodies, including less sharply discriminating sensory perception, which leads to poorer responsiveness in the appetite centers. But with the aid of additional mitochondria, all of these functions are actually raised back to, and in some cases beyond, what people experienced at a much tenderer age. And when it comes to weight loss, although many styles of yoga will calm down and slow the practitioner's metabolism *during the time that he or she is doing yoga*, the yoga will release PGC-1alpha. In the longer run, that induces mitochondrial proliferation. More mitochondria will convert more of what you eat into energy for your cells, accelerating fat metabolism.

TELOMERES

But there is still another way in which yoga helps with weight loss. In many instances, it actually turns back the clock. All creatures that are made up of more than one cell have strands of repetitive DNA protecting the precious DNA instructions that tell each cell what to be and what to do. Like bookends, these repetitive telomeres guard the special individual instruction-sets that make one egg a pigeon and another a trout. Each chromosome in each cell's nucleus has strings of telomeric DNA at both ends that stabilize these critical instruction-lists analogously to the way a tail stabilizes a kite in the wind. Generally, within generous limits, the longer the tail, the more stability.

The telomeres steady your DNA within the silent biochemical maelstrom that constitutes life in a cell. These telomeres are generally shortened by each cell division, so older cells are less stable, leading to all kinds of dysfunctional behavior of the DNA—from decreased immune-system specificity to increased incidence of cancer, from reduced thyroid hormone output to poorer digestion. One major way, in fact *the* major way, we age is explained by the shortening of telomeres.[11]

These telomeres appear to be the only aspect of inheritance that actually can be changed by what you do. The amount of stress in your life and how you handle it, what you eat, how active you are, and how happy you are may all affect telomere length, and may be passed on to your children. Your social support system, the trust you have in your friends and associates at work, even the neighborhood you live in can change the length of the telomeres in the DNA you pass on.

Although there are not yet any studies specifically targeting hatha yoga and telomeres, the practice of yoga, along with tai chi and qigong, has been shown to cut down on inflammation and oxidative stress—activities that are known to shorten telomeres. Further, meditation—whether in Jon Kabat-Zinn's mindfulness, Deepak Chopra's mantra-rich meditation retreats, or the more classical meditation generally practiced in the United States—actually increases *telomerase*, the enzyme that near-miraculously *adds* telomeres to your chromosomes.[12]

All of these practices have also been shown to shift gene expression away from stress and inflammatory reactions within cells. These effects reduce telomere loss and, in some cases, actually add to the telomeres on the DNA in the cell's nucleus.[13]

There is another charming aspect of telomeres: You don't have to fast for a week or complete arduous tasks of any kind to achieve lengthening. On the contrary, telomere length is increased by leisure activities, by lowering your stress, by doing things that make you happy.

In their book *The Telomere Effect*, Nobelist Elizabeth Blackburn and her colleague Elissa Epel define a person's "healthspan" as the number of years that person's cells are proliferating well, guided by longer strings of telomeres, and therefore consisting of essentially healthy tissues.[14] "Diseasespan," they write, is characterized by the years of illness and degeneration generally found in people at the far end of life. These authors argue extremely cogently that reduction in telomere length is one of the decisive factors in the transition from good health to chronic and terminal disease. When it comes to immune-system function, renewing your skin and the lining of your digestive tract, short-term memory, and even sexual prowess, telomere length is well correlated with youthful performance. The longer your telomeres, the more extensive your "healthspan." Yes, longevity itself is actually also more or less proportional to telomere length.

Discovering telomerase, the near-magical molecule that promotes telomere growth, won Blackburn the Nobel Prize. It has been proved that telomerase can actually increase the number of telomeres dangling from the ends of chromosomes. What would you think might promote that? Generally, the answer is lower stress, a positive attitude, and, yes, physical activities such as yoga. It has been proved that people who respond to difficult situations with pessimism, hostility, or feelings of inadequacy have statistically significantly shorter telomeres. Those who are optimistic and confident, rising to the challenges of adversity, activate their telomerase and lengthen their telomeres, even in times of stress.

Meditation is a critical aspect, indeed *the* critical aspect, of yogic life. Even without a detailed discussion I can certainly say it is well-documented common sense that meditation yields a less anxious person, and lowering anxiety aids in the loss of weight.[15] This has been proved at the biochemical level. As we have seen already, this applies to the metabolic machinery of every one of our billions of cells, to the tips of the chromosomes that foretell our longevity, and also at the feet-on-the-scale level.[16]

And now is a good time to summarize again the tangible ways yoga helps you lose weight. Neurophysiologically, yoga cuts down on your appetite by stretching the gastrointestinal tract, where receptors relay inhibitory signals to the appetite centers in the brain. And subtly, the foods that appeal to you may change; the apple may look more appetizing than the sausage.

Doing yoga helps you produce more burnable brown fat cells and cuts down on the more difficult-to-remove white fat cells. It induces your cells to have more mitochondria, increasing your overall metabolism.

And, as I must emphasize, yoga gives you calm, a way to reduce stress. This stress, the everyday kind you witness when a teacher is late for her class or traffic stops you from getting where you need to go, mobilizes hormones such as norepinephrine that actually accelerate oxidation in parts of cells, leading to degeneration. This is never desirable. But by providing the right sort of activity, yoga seems to promote and actually produce telomerase, improving your body's function.

CHAPTER 6

Motivation, Medical Risks, Drugs, and Diets

A RECENT STUDY FINDS that motivation for a given goal grows stronger as additional goals are linked to it. For example, a person will work harder and longer after realizing that more income will help send the children to college or even pay for that new couch.[1] Nathan Pritikin and Dean Ornish, MD, ushered in their groundbreaking diets beginning in the 1970s. Now, thanks to them, it's accepted that diet and exercise improve not just your figure but your health. That means cardiac health, which is affected by weight. But somewhat remarkably, living long enough to meet your great-grandchildren, looking cool, avoiding diabetes and heart disease, and staving off arthritis have provided *insufficient incentive* for greater and greater percentages of the population. This is a stunning, almost incomprehensible failure of motivation. I think it's urgent to find ways to help motivate anyone whose health may be affected by weight to take steps to correct the situation. What goals could one sensibly attach to weight loss that would make it appear worthwhile?

I write this believing that with its integral and unifying benefits to body and mind and therefore to spirit, yoga can increase some people's motivation over the threshold to the point where they take positive action. I have heard it said in New York that "even the religious no longer believe in God." Not being an expert on that, I take no position, but my personal experience and the experience of my students have shown me that the clearly nonsectarian but palpable spirituality of yoga will enhance the perceptions, clarify the thoughts, make more reasonable the attitudes, and pervade one's entire life. Religious or not, if you are reading this you are alive, and with or without the aid of the world's great faiths, personal spiritual elevation is more than just a joy. In an immediate and profound sense, I believe that yoga offers to you more life than is lived without it.

Yoga brings with it something that neither the purely secular slimming programs nor the traditional faiths can give you: a harmonizing of the body with the mind, and out of this union a growing sense, a somewhat aesthetic sense, that is also spiritual. It refines what you think of yourself, transcending the entirely secular "You are what you eat," with something closer to the Buddha's aphoristic observation that everything is connected and to B.K.S. Iyengar's proud pronouncement "Your body is your temple." The simple dignity of yoga combines with proven physiologic benefits to bring an apprehension of the sanctity of real life—each and every part of our very human bodies and minds.

So the overall objective is clear: to raise motivation to the boiling point, to the level at which action is irresistible. Yoga promises to add an overall transcendence, a depth of appreciation, and an elevation of awareness, all of which enhance many aspects of your personal life, including your associations with people and the natural world. All of this brings freedom to heed your own thoughts and intentions and to face your fears. Maybe above all, yoga helps you actually listen to yourself, mind and body, and also to your fellow beings. It is an additional, overall, even holy resonance with your body, which is part of the physical, mental, and spiritual practice of yoga. Let us marshal as many persuasive forces as possible to help you reach and remain at near-ideal body weight and mental lightness. Being a physician, I cannot fight off the urge to start with the medical inducements to moderation.

Weight preferences are quite different in various parts of the world and across the centuries. In sixteenth-century Holland, and in Jamaica today, bigger is more beautiful. We're inclined to say, *Chacun à son goût*, "There is no accounting for taste." But in century twenty-one, we cannot view our bodies as paintings hanging in a gallery to be passively and subjectively assessed while our minds remain stubbornly aloof and immutable. Our bodies are not separate from our minds. No, the aesthetic distance between them is no greater than that from our eyes to the mirror or to the numbers on the scale. We are changing parts of a changing world, living with one another, with our self-conscious impression of who each one of us is, and is becoming. And science has a lot to say about that.

WHY BEING OVERWEIGHT IS MEDICALLY DISCOURAGED

Most of us do not need to be told that weighing too much or too little isn't healthy, any more than we need a picture of a skull and crossbones on a cigarette package declaring that its contents are dangerous. It is not just a pun that overweight is a health epidemic of growing proportions. The point cannot be made strongly enough. But let me try.

DIABETES

Ninety percent of the almost 26 million diabetic Americans are overweight. This is a rough estimate, because demographic studies indicate that at least 7 million people have diabetes and do not know it. Approximately 95 percent of all diabetics have type 2 diabetes.[2] Obesity is a major independent risk factor for developing the disease, and more than 90 percent of type 2 diabetics are overweight or obese.[3] The relationship between being overweight and having type 2 diabetes is so intimate that as little as a 5 percent reduction in total body weight can improve type 2 diabetes in overweight or obese patients.[4]

Diabetes is a leader in the medical causes of amputations, blindness, and kidney failure and is a proven close associate of hypertension, stroke, retinal disease, coronary artery disease, neuropathy, complicated pregnancies, dental problems, and some forms of leukemia.[5] In fact, obesity even *impedes the treatment* of certain leukemias and melanoma.[6] A person with diabetes has twice the mortality risk of a similar-aged person without diabetes.[7] Diabetes itself is the seventh-greatest cause of mortality in the United States. In Europe, increases in blood-sugar levels beyond 100 milligrams per deciliter are correlated in a nearly linear fashion with increased death from all causes.[8]

Then there is prediabetes, which is obviously a red flag and is obviously also linked to overweight. Estimates range from 59 to 79 million Americans, and half of us over sixty-five years of age have prediabetes.

ARTHRITIS

When your belt size goes from 26 to 36, the dimensions of your foot, ankle, knee, and hip joints hardly budge. So the distribution of your weight, the stress per square inch, on these anatomical structures, your joints, grows right along with your overall size; it increases the same way the numbers on the scale do. One in five Americans have arthritis, but one in three overweight Americans have arthritis.

People who weigh more than is good for them have a worse time and an inferior outcome after conservative treatments for arthritis, and do not do as well after surgery either. The reason might be that some of the biochemicals associated with overweight seem to promote inflammation. A British study suggests that "excess adipose tissue produces humoral factors, altering articular cartilage metabolism," a more basic level of overweight-induced disrepair, specifically affecting the joints.[9]

Inflammation known to initiate and aggravate arthritis runs wilder in the systems of the overweight and obese, increasing both the arthritis and the pain it brings to its unfortunate victims. This is because overweight, and especially obesity, raises humoral factors in the blood and interstitial tissues that decrease production of PGC-1alpha, the potent anti-inflammatory that your body makes.[10] Lower PGC-1alpha, as discussed earlier, will stunt the mitochondrial population as well, inhibiting the proper functioning of all your cells, including the ones that make and sustain bone and cartilage.

As natural as water, PGC-1alpha reduces many other disease conditions as well. We will return to it when we consider the benefits of yoga; here we must focus on arthritis, citing the British study confirming that osteoarthritis of the knee is closely associated with

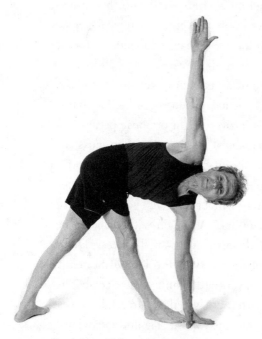

Parivrtta Trikonasana, the Twisted Triangle

weight, and so is the arthritis that is the hallmark of gout, again mentioning the humoral factors at a more profound level than just the physical factor of increased pressure on the joint.[11]

RECOVERY FROM SURGERY

It is entirely appropriate to list postsurgical recovery just after arthritis, because that's where arthritis, particularly when aggravated by the increased stress of overweight, makes things difficult. When it comes to the ever-more-popular total knee-replacement surgery, pain and disability are, with a few exceptions, also proportional to one's weight. The more overweight one is, the more likely knee surgery becomes, and the longer and more painful is the recovery from it. Yet overweight can sometimes be an advantage. Cardiac surgery is actually harder on the very thin, and mortality is lower as weight rises, but certain plastic-surgical procedures are twelve times more likely to have complications if the patient is obese.[12]

HEART DISEASE

Obesity is defined as a body mass index over 30. A person who is 5'8" tall and weighs 200 and a person who is 5'4" and weighs over 175 are in this category. These are rather extreme cases, but there has been a lot of research on them because they consume so much of our national healthcare resources. Information on them is indicative of the risk to other people who weigh more than their healthiest level but still not enough to qualify for this extreme label.

Obese people have an increased risk of developing vascular disease, sleep apnea, pulmonary hypertension, stroke, coronary artery disease, congestive heart failure, and arrhythmias, and are at increased risk of sudden death. Obese patients are six times more likely to have hypertension than lean patients.

"Fat-but-fit" is an illusion: Those overweight people who jog a great deal (though there may not be that many) *are* better off than those who don't, but they still have twice the chance of a serious cardiac event as their slimmer running buddies. As a country doctor once said, "Some people dig their graves with a knife and fork."

MOOD

But there is one other aspect of overweight that may be the most relevant of all: despair. No one knows whether the lopsided statistical preponderance of despair in the overweight is due to the medical complications, to distinct biochemical or mechanical effects of increased weight, or to the mild but pervasive societal stigma attached to extreme obesity. Naturally, there may be other factors. Then there are both sides of the chicken and egg: Does deep depression cause obesity, or do things go the other way around? Maybe it's just feeling out of it and out of place in our culture, which seems to worship thinness.

But whatever its cause, despair is a passive thing. You "fall into despair," or "experience despair." No one gets up, goes out, and despairs. Overweight is strongly associated with despair.[13] And weight is something you can take into your own hands. But, admittedly, despair makes it harder.

From extensive clinical experience and reading the current literature, I'm sure there is no reason on earth that you cannot lose any amount of weight you want to lose. Trying and succeeding substantially reduces the sense of helplessness, and that cuts directly into despair. Losing unwanted weight is the opposite of a vicious circle: It is "Nothing succeeds like success." Overweight does cause illness, there is no doubt, but overweight is also associated with unhappiness, even controlling for other factors such as medical conditions and pain.[14] You can beat this game, get out of the dysfunctional cycle of eating, feeling bad, eating more, and feeling worse. If you are so moved, I invite you to try.

OTHER OPTIONS

Before actually going over more of the yoga that is so likely to help, and so unlikely to cause you an iota of harm, we must review the alternatives to yoga.

DRUGS

There are a huge number of medications for weight loss. That fact, by itself, suggests that this type of treatment is still not satisfactory. Although chemically they are quite a varied lot, essentially, we can categorize them as either of two types: One group affects a number of different systems; for instance, amphetamines cut down appetite and speed up metabolism. The other group has just one effect on one system that is meant to slow down or reverse the whole process of gaining weight. The first group is like taking steroids away from a football player: He gets smaller muscles and has less energy. The second group's modus operandi is comparable to slowing down one conveyor belt on a production line: The whole factory's output will decline.

The advantage of medications in the first, systemic group is that they might have meager effects on a number of bodily systems, and therefore are less severe in their side effects. The disadvantage is that by affecting many systems, they might profoundly alter quality of life. The advantage of the single-effect group is that overall life is not affected, but the disadvantage is that the one aspect that the drug works on may be changed quite a bit.

The system-affecting group: One medication, approved in 2016, is Qsymia, a timed-release combination of the classical weight-losing, appetite-inhibiting, metabolism-increasing phentermine, and topiramate, a medicine used to tame seizures and curb migraine headaches. The phentermine is an amphetamine-like molecule, which has a well-deserved reputation for causing adverse neurological effects such as paraesthesias, dizziness, insomnia, and altered sense of taste, as well as more standard side effects: constipation and dry mouth. But these are just the most common side effects. Fetal harm, diarrhea, psychomotor retardation, poor concentration and memory, and jaundiced eyes are among many, many others.[15]

We have already reviewed the "adverse effects" of overweight. Exchanging one set of these effects for another may not be progress. The FDA generally approves drugs that are as good as or better than others that perform the same function. The fact that the FDA has recently approved a medication with this kind of profile gives us a hint about the quality and safety of the older weight-loss medications.

Suprenza is another phentermine medication. Minus the side effects due to topiramate, the story is the same. Not to overstate the case, side effects may include dizziness, dry mouth, trouble sleeping (insomnia), irritability, nausea, vomiting, diarrhea, constipation, restlessness, euphoria, feeling uneasy, difficulty breathing, weakness, swelling of the ankles and feet, increased blood pressure, fatigue, headache, unpleasant taste in the mouth, changes in sex drive, or impotence.[16]

Saxenda is different. It is a GLP-1 receptor agonist (a glucagon-like protein), which has a much broader physiological influence on the body. To make a long story short, it works on different bodily systems to reduce appetite, keeping blood sugar high so that the body craves less food and slowing the stomach's release of food for digestion by the intestine. These and other factors reduce appetite.

This is particularly interesting because, as described in chapter 3, yoga does the same thing in a different way: It coaxes the body into acting as though it has just finished a satisfying meal by stimulating the stretch receptors in the digestive tract. But Saxenda has side effects that you may not savor: In rodent test-subjects, it caused benign and malignant thyroid tumors. In people, it is also associated with thyroid tumors, suicidal behavior and ideation, hypoglycemia, and the almost inevitable trio of diarrhea/nausea/vomiting.[17] Yoga, of course, has no such side effects. Rather, it has been used to treat many of these conditions.

Contrave is a combination of an antidepressant (bupropion) and an opioid antagonist (naltrexone). Chemically it is a fairly close relative of amphetamine, but it also has a nicotinic effect, and it is sometimes used as a quit-smoking medication. It goes to work on the central nervous system, and its side effects may then appear: suicidal behavior and thoughts (which, given overweight's association with despair, is particularly ominous), heightened risk of seizure, hypertension and tachycardia, psychosis and delusion, hostility, anxiety and panic, liver damage (from the naltrexone), angle-closure glaucoma (due to the antidepressant), and hypoglycemia.[18]

Single-action medications: One medicine that targets a single function is Xenical. It works in a novel way by binding with enzymes in the stomach and intestine that break down fats and just keeping you from digesting fats. This prevents fatty substances from passing out of your intestine and into your bloodstream. One good feature of the drug is that it acts in such a limited sphere. Xenical targets the food in your stomach and the enzymes that digest it, rather than any of the systems or cells in the rest of your body. But in order to be effective, Xenical has to have a pretty strong effect on those enzymes. It is no surprise that taking it leads to frequent oily stools, oily spotting, intestinal gas with discharge, and sometimes poor bowel control.[19]

That is enough about these medicines. You must evaluate the pros and cons, and consider them in competition with yoga.

Meds versus happiness: The critical decision of whether to lose weight, gain weight, or forget about it altogether and go to the movies, lies with the elusive bluebird of happiness. A British study of 163,066 individuals found, as we have amply demonstrated already, that poor health goes along with overweight, and that in men unhappiness is correlated strongly with poor health. In women health declined as weight rose, as with the men, but women were also unhappier as their overall weight increased, *independent* of their individual health status.[20]

When you look at the literature relating to all of these medicines, one thing stands out. In each case, the prescribing information requires that patients who take the drug do so with a low-calorie diet and exercise. So whichever medication the patient leaves the doctor's office with, it's pretty certain that dietary measures and exercise are part of what they've been advised to take up.

DIETS: An ulterior motive lies behind parading all the dangers of overweight before a reader prone to despair. If you hear exactly the right number of horrible things about overweight—not so few as to allow you to shrug them off and not so many that they only deepen remorse and despondency—you just might act. What follows is a further attempt to give you even better reasons for doing what you already want to do. It also affirms that yoga is a safe and effective way to do it.

Still, any alternative program for losing weight must acknowledge a great debt to two brave clinical researchers. They focused more on cardiovascular disease and revolutionized the treatment for it and for overweight, one of its chief causes. I am thinking of Nathan Pritikin and Dean Ornish, MD.

Nathan Pritikin began his professional life as an engineer, and may have begun pondering cardiac disease in terms of input-output systems. He developed a rigorous exercise and strict dietary program of strategically low fats, and managed to help most people following his program reverse cardiac arterial disease. Dean Ornish did essentially the same thing by emphasizing a low-stress approach to life that features meditation and yoga. The two of them have revolutionized medical care and drawn our attention to more prosaic aspects of our lives that they proved quite rigorously to be medically relevant.

The current attention to gluten, GMOs, supplements, the paleo diet, the Mito diet, the Whole30 diet, and indeed (to some extent) yoga began with these two men. Appropriate diet and just about any safe exercise are compatible and synergic with the ideas and the actual yoga in this book. Eventually, with better understanding of the human genome, these dietary recommendations may be specifically made for individuals. For now, they are general recommendations at best.

Caloric reduction and the yo-yo effect: Most people trumpeting the wonders of their diets end up right back where they started, at pre-diet levels—in two to three years.

There are some reasons for the yo-yo effect that aren't completely obvious. According to National Institutes of Health researcher Kevin Hall, people who lose weight typically keep it off for a while, then plateau and later regain those pounds.[21] When we begin a weight-loss program, we often make radical changes in the way we eat—for instance, absolutely no carbs, or absolutely no sugar. These alterations in diet are usually very difficult to maintain, and slowly we begin to reintroduce those things we were so eager to cut out, under the illusion that if we don't add too much we won't gain back the pounds we shed. For instance, after eating very little or no bread for a few months, you might feel that treating yourself to a slice or two won't hurt. They won't, if you eat them one time. If you add them back into your diet regularly, you will see the results when you step on the scale.

Then there is calorie counting. Food labels often underestimate or inaccurately state the number of calories the foods contain. So even those who carefully count the calories they take in might be making some mistakes.[22]

Even more important is the difference between how one's body digests protein and carbohydrate, how one's body loses or keeps processed foods and natural ones. Though these foods may have the same caloric content, they may be stored or used differently. And even without counting calories, we must consider that our genes do have an impact on our weight. Researchers are studying whether people inherit the risk for overweight, and the answer is a resounding yes. Obesity-risk scores may even predict how much weight a high-risk person can expect to carry.[23]

On top of all that, we are just beginning to become aware of how the bacteria in our gut can influence our health in general and our weight in particular; more research is needed. How we prepare food, whether we eat at home or in restaurants, how much we exercise, how much or how little we sleep, and how long and how deeply we are happy or sad also influence both weight loss and gain.

Fortunately, we are beginning to count calories less and look at the types of foods we eat more. A consistent diet of unprocessed foods and plenty of fruits and vegetables, along with exercise, is likely to result in more stable weight with fewer downs followed by ups.

Although we are trying to leave the medications behind, diet pills have been around for a long time. Many are biochemically sophisticated. Some activate the "fat-burning hormone" (leptin), reversing the usual trend. Generally, the medicines alter bodily functions, and the bodily functions affect what you eat, as, for example, amphetamines change activity in your brain, and that affects what you eat. While diet pills may appear to be effective, at least at first, almost all have undesirable side effects that discourage continued use. An example on the frontier between medicine and diet is supplements that contain extracts of the South Asian fruit *Garcinia cambogia*. This is supposed to suppress appetite and increase serotonin (the "happy chemical") secretion and therefore is supposedly quite appropriate for "emotional eaters." However, these supplements can have negative side effects, such as headache and dizziness. A medical journal article concluded that, while more research is necessary, these supplements don't really help with weight loss. Further, *Garcinia cambogia* also may cause liver necrosis, a malady that can prove fatal.[24]

Other weight-reduction programs do not necessarily include the important element of exercise but go directly to one point: Those who wish to lose weight must focus on taking in fewer calories. Essentially, there are three other ways to curtail consumption, and yoga is compatible with all three. Used together, they are synergistic.

1. Mindfulness beyond the menu. Eating *seriously*, by which I mean *not* reading the paper or fooling with your cell phone, but slowing down significantly and feeling the texture and the warmth or coldness, and smelling and tasting the flavors of what you eat, will help you feel satisfied sooner. Simply paying attention to the process of eating—being alert to the process of food selection, preparation, and ingestion—can do a lot to make you significantly more satisfied earlier in your meals, whether you are at home or out.

2. Whole lifestyle shift: changing the way you feel about eating in general, so you end up eating less. This might begin, for example, by noticing that we are moving parts of a delicate planet, with 7.8 billion large mammals eating and excreting every day. Each one of our 7.8×10^9 contributions makes a difference. Seeking harmony in what we buy, what we eat, and what we give back to Earth is something we can do to improve things.

3. Altering what you eat through diet. The Whole30 does this in a consciously self-limiting way, asking you to refrain from sugar, alcohol, grains, dairy, legumes, peanut butter, carrageenan, MSG, sulfites, and baked or junk food for thirty days. Other diets do it by giving you either meals, calorie counts, do's and don'ts, or a point system.

The more elemental diets work with the basic food groups and promote low-carbohydrate, high-protein meals (Atkins, paleo, Mito, keto), some of which actually stimulate mitochondria, which is a good thing; others have specially prepared meals that are guaranteed to take off one or two pounds every week (e.g., the Hyperfit diet), or give you shakes, bars, and tidbits that will help (e.g., SlimFast). Others, such as Medifast and Nutrisystem, give you a small number of alternative meals delivered to your home.

There are diets for vegans, for example, Vegan Diet, and many diets for diabetics, the people who may need them the most. I recommend the Diabetes Diet in Dr. Richard Bernstein's book of the same name. Dietitians and nutritionists can also design a food plan that is right for you as an individual. A number of them recommend meals that are nutritious and have balanced vitamins and electrolytes. One book matches your ideal dietary composition to your blood type: *Eat Right for Your Type.*

Weight Watchers may be in a class by itself, using a point system for foods you eat rather than counting calories. Working on motivation, employing peer pressure and group support meetings, Weight Watchers furnishes thousands of recipes and presents a strong history of success. No side effects, no extra risks. This program has helped several people I know, one of whom had been overweight since she was a toddler.

So, in summary, diets must be praised for their ability to show you that your weight is in your hands. Many people have discovered to their delight that they can modify their weight with diets. On the negative side of the ledger, unfortunately, the weight lost through even the most gradual, thoughtful diet is almost invariably regained. Dieting can be done with low or high motivation, but in itself, a diet supplies no motive for its own pursuit or continuation. Therein lies its greatest difference from yoga.

SURGERY

A third weight-loss strategy involves reducing the volume of your stomach. The surgeon cuts part of it away and either sews up a smaller pouch with what remains or, using a more recently developed technique, inserts balloons that take up space that would otherwise be occupied by food. In the cutting option, the surgeon has to be careful not to remove too many of the receptors and enterocrine glands that limit appetite; I believe the balloon techniques are still too new to evaluate.

All these methods alter either what and how much you eat or how well you digest. None approaches the act of eating itself, or the underlying motivation and other pressures associated with the activity. This is yoga's greatest strength.

I met Marcie Hammond when I worked with the people at Beachbody. Marcie is a forty-seven-year-old wardrobe assistant in the company's video-filming unit who not only believes yoga has helped her to lose many pounds but says it has saved her life.

How much did I weigh when I started doing yoga? 205. I'd been a yo-yo dieter; two years ago I lost sixty-two pounds. Put half back after two years. Then depression, menopause. When I went into menopause I gained fifty pounds. I've always lost and gained all my life. I never knew why I was losing and gaining. I felt like I was losing it in my body but not in my mind. A lot of weight gain is emotional. Not physical. When we fall into depression, or stressing, we emotionally eat. That's what's been going on in me all my life.

Yoga is a different approach for me. I went into it because I was broken, depressed, couldn't keep going on. I thought it was only for skinny people, flexible people. I never knew I could do it until Beachbody's three-week yoga program. With yoga you get the tranquility. It helps mentally. This was my last resort. I felt like I was at the end of the road, like I could fall and never get up again.

Because of what I had lost two years before and then gained back I felt like a failure, like a liar. So I started doing yoga. Very intimidating. I couldn't do any of the moves, but I could do the modified part. I couldn't do full stretches. The instructor taught for three weeks. We were doing it at home with DVDs and had three classes a week. I felt different than I've ever felt with any weight-loss program, with anything. I was targeting the problem part in my life, concentrating on my mind and spirit. Doing that, taking care of my body. Seeing results. Wanting to eat even healthier.

We were also on a food plan. Eating healthy, doing my yoga, getting my mind together. I was able to adjust my antidepressant, to lower the dose. I felt I could sleep better. I was more focused. I was breathing better. I learned how to relax. And so, now, after five months I'm still doing yoga.

Yoga is my life now because if I don't do it I can't go through my day. It's like my new medicine. I have to deal with the day, do my yoga in the morning, and sometimes I also do it at night. It keeps me controlled physically and mentally. Also I want to keep weight off. Hope.

It's the answer to my life's questions: emotional eating, menopause, insomnia. Yoga came right on time.

As of today I've lost fifty-five pounds. Every Monday morning I weigh myself and see how I am. Depends on everything—you need to keep tabs on what you're doing.

I was a junk-food addict. Healthy food isn't easy for me to eat, but I know it's a necessity, and I need to learn to incorporate it and enjoy it. I see the benefits of it. I can't deprive myself seven days a week or I get depressed and binge. That's not healthy. So I give myself a reward one day a week. I don't punish myself.

Meditation came with yoga. That helps me. I stop when I feel uncomfortable, breathe and meditate and it works wonders for me. I don't eat or pop a pill. I wish I had found this years ago. I looked at those thin, young pretzels, I felt like I couldn't be like them. But I'm more flexible now than I've ever been in my life. Emotional eating and menopause, many of us have problems with it. I was focusing on physical but needed to focus on mental too.

CHAPTER 7

Doing the Yoga

YOGA WILL GIVE YOU reverence for the world—make you see it and appreciate it more. It will give you the same benefit when it comes to your own body. This will silently, maybe even without your awareness, bring about cumulative, titanic changes in your life. The first small shifts in the way you feel and see the world will lead to greater adaptive changes. I say this unreservedly, both as a man with a forty-some-year daily yoga practice and as a physician who has observed many patients over a long period of time. Yoga is theistic but nonsectarian. It has codes of living that are eerily similar to the Ten Commandments.[1] Like many religions, yoga brings about an elevated and liberated sense of reality. But yoga has no clergy of any kind, and no initiation rite or fee: To be a yogi is to do yoga. That's all. It is as simple as that. Yoga has spiritual origins, and spiritual goals, but you cannot plausibly profess yogic beliefs without doing yoga. Yoga is linked to your mental and bodily actions during the day; it helps you sleep at night. But its basic thrust is spiritual.

This may be yoga's greatest argument against weighing too much. It promotes realization of your own sanctity. It distinguishes what is pleasant from what is good, giving you potent motivation to seek what is good for you, and to stay away from what is not good. This much it has in common with every spiritual enterprise. But yoga necessarily involves your bodily actions. It leaves you with allegiance to nothing but what is good for you and the world, and the energy and preferences to pursue it. You must *do* yoga!

The most reasonable place to start is with the human anatomy and physiology that we covered in chapter 5. A number of yoga poses stretch the abdomen and its contents, as we have said. The stretch receptors in the first part of the small intestine (the duodenum), in the stomach, and in the last part of the esophagus have direct connection with the appetite centers in the brain. Anatomically speaking, the tenth cranial nerve, the vagus nerve, has sensory fibers that gather in signals and send them up to the brain's nucleus solitarius, which connects to parts of the hypothalamus, the nucleus accumbens, and the arcuate nucleus, which greatly influence the impulse to eat. When the stretch receptors are aroused (by expanding the stomach through the increase in the volume of its contents, or through the stretch of yoga poses), appetite is curtailed. There are specific yoga poses that take advantage of these anatomical facts.

It makes sense to start with the simplest poses that are the easiest to do well, and move up to the more advanced versions when you feel it is safe to do so. You will be learning the dignified and elegant workings of your body, *from the inside*, and simultaneously doing poses that can curb your caloric intake. With this rare but natural union, you will see the sanctity of your body and mind, and shed a spiritual light on your life.

BASIC GROUND RULES FOR DOING YOGA

- Read over each pose and look at the photos before attempting it.
- Practice in a softly lit, level, clean, safe place.
- Relax to improve receptivity and extend self-control.
- Work with a teacher if possible so that, if you are unfamiliar with yoga, you can begin by knowing you are doing the poses correctly.
- Learn as much of the relevant anatomy as you can.
- Visualize the stretch receptors sending signals to tamp down the impulse to eat. Visualizing what is happening inside as well as outside your body when you do the postures can be a valuable tool, just as knowing the streets of a city helps you get from place to place.
- Do each pose one time—give it a good try, then move on. No reason to obsess; next time you'll have another chance to do better.
- Think of the person or people you've loved the most in your life. Be as kind to yourself as you would be to them.

- Rest for five to fifteen minutes after doing the full set of postures, whenever possible. Always get one to two minutes of highly concentrated rest.
- Do the poses on an empty or emptyish stomach.
- Wait at least three hours after eating before doing yoga, and four or even five hours after eating if you have gastric reflux or are over fifty-five years of age.

To proceed, please read the contraindications to make sure you can do the pose. The contraindications (except as noted) are almost all relative. If you have a contraindicated condition, an experienced and resourceful teacher can find a similar or related pose with the same benefits for most people in most cases. Almost invariably a simpler version, a version using props, or another type of work-around will serve the same purpose.[2] Once learned, these poses are most effective if done fifteen to thirty minutes before a meal, even if you learn the poses in class or at another time of day.

The commonly useful props are a yoga mat, a belt, and a block. Card-table chairs or chairs of similar construction are also valuable at times.

Don't push your body to the point where there is severe pain or even severe discomfort. While yoga can heal, it is also possible to injure yourself. A little discomfort may be okay (though be careful). The goal of yoga is to gain control, not lose it. If pain occurs, stop the pose and see a good yoga teacher or physician. If you have begun with easier variations, move up toward the classical pose when you are able.

ASANA

All the poses here are helpful for weight loss, but each person will find him- or herself better suited for some than for others. As you begin practicing, you want to find the poses that are right for you. The best tip-off may be the contraindications. They come before the directions for each pose and list the conditions for which that pose is not advisable. Begin with the poses that have no good reason for you *not* to go into them fully. The benefits rise as your inhibitions fall.

Play to your strengths, but also respect your needs. If you're very flexible, the backbends are made for you. If your main concern is overeating at lunch, then you'll likely be doing the poses at work, and standing postures may be the only way to go. If balance is an issue, start with the seated poses. Take care of alignment first, then do the postures vigorously. Doing the poses fifteen to thirty minutes before eating, doing them consistently for three to four weeks—that's what works. Weigh yourself before and after that period of time. When the number on the scale gets lower, it will help your confidence that this is something you can do, and something that's effective. I hope you will enjoy this, because in so many ways yoga—if you let it—will be a valuable and trustworthy lifelong companion.

Many yoga poses have more than one proven benefit. For example, forward bends are good for spinal stenosis, and also for tight hamstrings. When there is a significant benefit that is largely applicable, it is mentioned below in the write-up of the pose. After you have learned a good many poses, these other benefits may help you select which poses you do on any given day.

STANDING

Sometimes standing is the best you can do:

1. With hip arthritis, after total hip replacement (posterior approach), herniated lumbar disc, piriformis syndrome; or when the only place to do yoga is in a washroom
2. When other circumstances leave you unable to sit

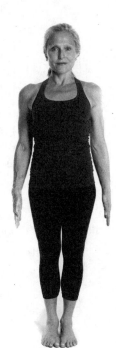

Tadasana, the Mountain

Tadasana
The Mountain

Which yoga practitioner cannot recall an early class in which he or she was asked to stand, well balanced, sturdy and alert, in this pose, imitating the living tranquility of an immovable mountain? Who has not stood, nearly tingling with a newfound sense of attentive calm, conscious of the body's sheath of skin and of the powerful, even surge of internal, attentive calm? The sense of self is undeniable, particularly as one does not stir.

Benefits and how it works: Exemplifies the magical joys of simple self-discipline. Motionlessness slows the breath, and begins a cascade of physical and mental calm. The pose fosters good posture, self-reliance, and a sense of individuality, as well as the joy and responsibility of having a body in the first place.

Contraindications: Flexion contractures of the foot, ankle, knees, or hips; major leg-length discrepancy; severe imbalance; advanced congestive heart failure or chronic venous insufficiency.

THE POSE

1. Stand with your feet facing forward, as wide apart as your hips.
2. Raise your toes and spread them out, then place them down, increasing the territory on which you are standing.
3. Sense the floor with the slender stems of your toes: the thinner parts between your foot and the toes' pulpy last segments.
4. Divide your weight into twelve parts for each foot: Place six on each heel, two for each big toe, and one for each of the other toes and related metatarsal heads.
5. By adjusting your pelvis, shoulders, and neck, set your ankles, hips, shoulders, and ears in a plumb line.
6. Look straight ahead with calm, learning eyes.
7. Relax the soft and hard palates inside your mouth.
8. Get longer, especially at the nape of your neck and at the Achilles tendons.
9. Let the last digits of your fingers and thumbs be heavy enough to open your hands, taking tension off the cuticles.
10. Breathe slowly, quietly, and symmetrically: side to side, front to back, for at least a minute.

Vriksasana
The Tree

Benefits and how it works: Improves posture sufficiently to stretch the esophagus and more forward parts of the stomach itself. In this way it is a mild inhibitor of appetite. Accomplishing this elegantly simple pose—a matter of coordination, range of motion, and balance—gives a sense of self-reliance and confidence. It takes a little time to be solidly stable, but after mastering it, practitioners are delighted to assume this posture as a sign and proof of self-sufficiency and grace. In addition, it safely challenges and gradually improves balance. Further, the pose applies vertical and lateral pressure to the hip and spine, which stimulates osteocytes and strengthens bones. It enhances alertness, focus, and symmetry.

Contraindications: Grossly impaired balance, severe rotator cuff syndrome, plantar fasciitis, peroneal palsy, subacromial impingement, ankle instability.

Helpful hints: Distribute your weight firmly and securely on the standing foot: 50 percent on the heel, about 25 percent on the big toe and the other 25 percent divided equally among each of the lesser toes and metatarsal pads; look intently at a point level with your eyes; expand the front and sides of your rib cage as you raise your arms overhead, stretching them upward as far as possible.

THE CLASSIC POSE (VARIATIONS FOLLOW)

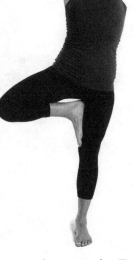

1. Stand with your feet hip-width apart, toes spread out. Press the ball and heel of your left foot firmly into the floor. Tighten the left quadriceps and hamstrings moderately, making the whole thigh firm. Advance the lower pelvis forward, which will mildly extend your hip. These maneuvers should reduce your lumbar curve.
2. Align your pelvis directly above your feet. Elevate and place your right foot at the root of your left thigh, close to where the limb joins the torso, toes pointing toward the left ankle. If your leg doesn't get up that high, place it lower on the thigh, or on the calf. Avoid placing it directly on the side of the knee.
3. Retain a forward-facing pelvis as you carefully swing the bent right knee and thigh out to the side (ideally at ninety degrees to the left foot).

Vriksasana, the Tree

4. If your right hip is now higher than the left, dip the right knee downward, stretching the quadriceps. That usually helps level the hips.

5. Reopen the hips by pressing the lower pelvis forward again. Refocus your gaze to a point at eye level, fifteen to twenty feet away.

6. Slowly inhale as you raise your arms symmetrically, turning the palms inward to meet above your head, biceps as far behind the ears as possible without jutting your head forward. Let your lungs fill completely as you do so.

7. Bring your shoulder blades close together behind you; stretch upward from your left ankle to your finger- and thumbtips. Stretch skyward; leave only the skin of the sole of your foot on the mat.

8. Take several slow, symmetrical breaths in and let even slower breaths out.

9. Then let your arms descend as you exhale.

10. Slowly repeat the cycle of arm elevation and breathing several times. Come out of the pose slowly, placing both feet squarely on the floor. Repeat, reversing your legs.

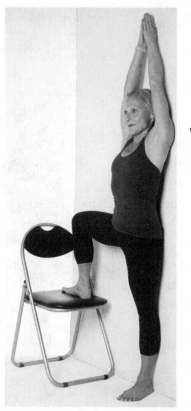

Vriksasana

VARIATIONS

1. Brace the side of a chair against a wall so it faces you when you stand with the chair to your right and with your back against the wall. Place your right foot on the seat of the chair, toes pointing away from you. Then proceed as above. This is a way to begin stretching the gastrointestinal tract, and a safe and sensible way to start challenging your balance on one foot. To do that gradually, lift your right foot somewhat, reducing the weight on it to the point of eventually lifting it off the chair. This is actually more difficult than the classical pose, but safer.

2. Do the pose against a wall but without a chair. Tuck the right heel into the root of the left

thigh, or onto the lower thigh or calf. This pose is still very safe.

The supporting of one leg by the other will probably tighten abdominal musculature and cause you to rebalance your posture all over again. Therein lies the inhibition of appetite.

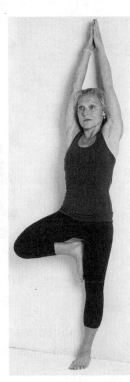

Vriksasana

Virabhadrasana I
Warrior I

Benefits and how it works: Produces a vertical arch of the back, stretching the distal esophagus, entire stomach, and duodenum, which will lessen appetite. It also reduces the pain of herniated lumbar or thoracic discs, as it creates a partial vacuum at the fronts of the vertebral bodies of the lumbar and thoracic spine, drawing herniated disc material forward. This returns the disc material to its proper place underneath the vertebral bodies and away from the nerve roots it would otherwise irritate.

Contraindications: Severe knee-joint derangement, especially anterior or posterior cruciate ligament pathology; plantar fasciitis; Achilles tendonitis; extreme weakness; central spinal stenosis.

THE POSE

1. Step or jump your legs four and a half feet apart, arms horizontal, palms up. Take two slow, deep breaths.
2. Turn the right foot ninety degrees outward and the left foot thirty degrees inward, as you raise your arms to vertical. With your legs straight, advance your left hip forward and your right hip back

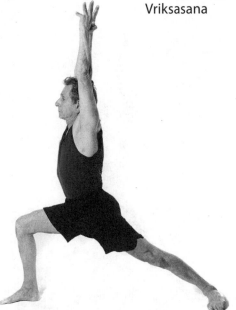

Virabhadrasana I, Warrior I

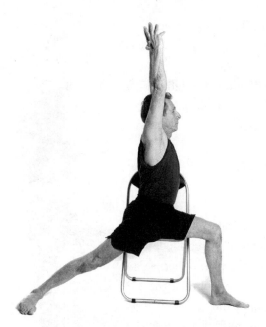

Virabhadrasana I—with chair for imbalance and/or weakness

ninety degrees until your navel faces straight forward.

3. Bend your right knee to a right angle, shin vertical, thigh horizontal. Rock some of your weight back to the ball of the big toe, outer arch, and heel of your left foot. Use the ball of your left foot to counter that force and retain the advance of the left hip.

4. Stretch your fingers and especially your thumbs up to the sky.

5. Breathe evenly for sixty seconds.

6. Return to standing by reversing the sequence. Then do all five steps with the left leg forward.

VARIATIONS

1. Bend your left leg and rest the thigh on a chair seat, parallel to the back of the chair. Place the right hand on the bent thigh; use the left for balance by holding the back of the chair. As you get more secure, gradually, over a week or more, raise yourself off the chair. Use your quadriceps, not your arms, to do this. Move your arms to your sides or even over your head as balance permits.

2. Place a block under the forward leg in the classical pose. This lifts the torso and rocks it backward, encouraging more extension of the lower lumbar spine, stretching the gastrointestinal

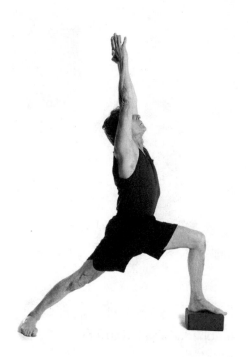

Virabhadrasana I—for tilted pelvis

tract, but also letting the less flexible spine come to vertical. A wider stance, in which the legs are not in a straight line, vitiates the therapeutic effects of this pose, but makes it a little easier.

BACKBENDS

Certainly the most exhilarating poses, and probably the most effective appetite suppressants. As it happens, these poses are also therapeutic for herniated discs, as explained in my book *Healing Yoga*, and are not recommended for people suffering from spinal stenosis, anterolisthesis, or facet syndrome.[3] Herniated discs are actually more common in people who are overweight, making these poses doubly effective for those individuals.

Pay attention to your alignment; it's crucial. As you practice, your body will adapt to these poses. Start out holding the poses for ten to twenty seconds, because they are arduous. Then gradually build up to a minute or even more.

Salabhasana
The Locust

Benefits and how it works: Stretches the anterior portions of the esophagus, stomach, and duodenum, curbing appetite by sending inhibiting signals to the nucleus solitarius and other appetite centers within the brain. Strengthens the extensor muscles of the entire spine.

For lower back pain due to a herniated disc, a common injury for those who may be carrying extra pounds: Creates a partial vacuum at the front of the disc by separating the anterior portions of the vertebrae above and below the disc. This sucks the herniated disc into alignment with the vertebrae, away from nerve roots as they exit the spine. Holding the pose will strengthen the quadratus lumborum, the multifidus, the iliocostalis, and other muscles that can arch the back and accomplish these two purposes.

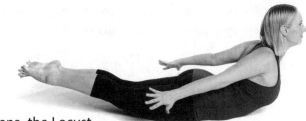

Salabhasana, the Locust

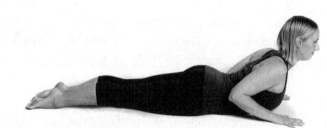

Salabhasana—raising intensity

Contraindications: GERD (gastric reflux), spinal stenosis, spondylolisthesis (anterolisthesis), facet syndrome, pregnancy in second or third trimesters.

THE POSE

1. Lie prone, arms at your sides with your palms down. Stretch out the front of your body from your forehead, your throat, your solar plexus just below your ribs, your hips, and the tops of your feet—down to your toes' cuticles.
2. Lift from your Adam's apple and the backs of your knees. Lift the nape of your neck and your Achilles tendons.
3. Gently pressing your ankles together, inhale and lift your arms parallel to the floor, palms down. Elongate your entire body, but especially the front.
4. Although somewhat counterintuitive, soften your stomach muscles. Tightening them only serves to reduce the arching here. You will get further and do better with the "flat tire" abdomen in this situation, and you will inhibit appetite still more.

LESS CHALLENGING VARIATION

Place your palms underneath your shoulders and press down to raise your torso. In this version, retain contact between the abdomen and the mat or floor. Be careful not to throw your head back too far. Raise your throat, not your forehead.

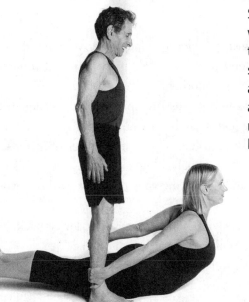

Salabhasana—one way to improve: Grasp the ankles of a teacher standing on tiptoes astride Salabhasana, and as far back as you can reach. Then the teacher lowers his heels.

Setu Bandhasana
The Bridge

Benefits and how it works: Stretches the lower chest, a postural improvement in itself, but also, by arching the thoracic and lumbar spine, it further stretches and elongates the esophagus, the stomach, and the duodenum. In addition, by flexing the cervical region, it holds the throat and adjacent upper esophagus in place, somewhat raising the tension on the lower esophagus, stomach, and duodenum.

Contraindications: GERD, herniated cervical disc, severe kyphosis, advanced arthritis, advanced pregnancy, lumbar spinal stenosis.

Setu Bandhasana, the Bridge

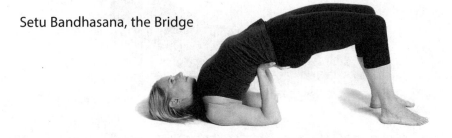

THE POSE

1. Lie on your back with a folded blanket under your shoulders but not under your head. Bend your knees and place your feet squarely on the floor and parallel to one another.
2. Use your quadriceps to put pressure on your feet, as though you were trying to push your feet away from you, but don't actually move your feet. Use the backward force of your legs to generate forward force that will lift your torso and pelvis higher, arching your back, elevating your pubic region, and advancing your chest forward over your throat as much as possible.
3. Support yourself with your hands under your lower back, elbows at right angles, fingers pointing toward each other.
4. Breathe slowly and carefully, filling your lungs from the back to the front: from their bottoms, near the diaphragm and kidneys, upward and forward toward the top ribs.
5. As you do this, push more on your feet, elevating your mid-torso and pubic region more, and bringing your chest up and toward vertical.
6. Relax the anal muscles and pelvic diaphragm to stretch the esophagus and stomach and duodenum even more, but always gently.
7. Remain in the pose for at least thirty seconds. A minute is better.

LESS CHALLENGING VARIATIONS (BLANKETS IN A SIMILAR POSITION)

1. Instead of actively lifting your torso, lie in the same position on bolsters, large pillows, or multiple blankets.
2. Place one or more blocks underneath your sacrum and lift from there.

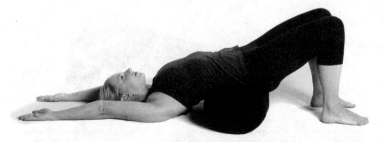

Setu Bandhasana, variation 1—with bolster for weakness

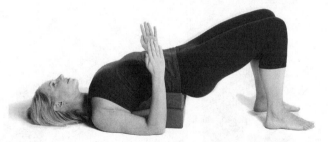

Setu Bandhasana, variation 2—with block for strengthening

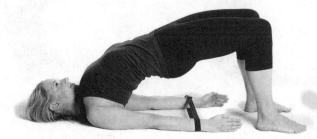

Setu Bandhasana, variation 3—with belt for improvement

3. Strap your elbows together so they are shoulder-distance apart. The strap goes around the arms above the elbows, but may be placed above the wrists. Lift your pelvis; you may place your hands underneath your lower back for support. This will also stretch the stomach across its entire girth.

Ustrasana
The Camel

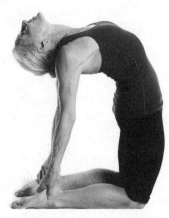

Benefits and how it works: This is a greater, all-inclusive stretch, and when done correctly, almost all your digestive tract is elongated. The small intestine zigzags crazily some twenty-eight feet in the abdomen, so do not worry that you will tear, snap, or fray anything; there is plenty of "slack." But the whole tract is loosely bound down in various places by structural connective tissue, called the omentum, and the gastroduodenal ligament, which holds the lower stomach and beginning of the duodenum in place, so some tension will definitely be created.

Ustrasana, the Camel

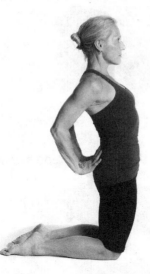

Ustrasana—early
beginner

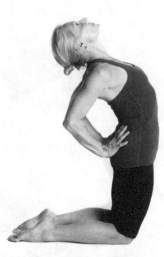

Ustrasana—
later beginner

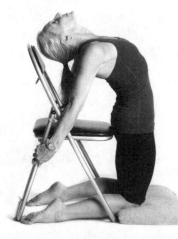

Ustrasana—
intermediate

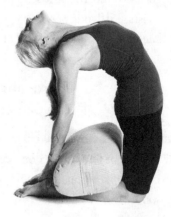

Ustrasana—with
delicate knees

For herniated disc: By arching the entire spine, a partial vacuum is formed between the front parts of the vertebral bodies, which draws the herniated disc material forward, away from the nerve fibers. Since the shortest distance between two points is a straight line, the global curve also works to slide the spinal cord upward through the vertebral canal, toward the head, enabling it to adjust to regions of compression.

Contraindications: Cervical vertebral displacement, spinal stenosis, anterolisthesis, anterior labral tear (hips), severe arthritis, carotid or vertebral arterial disease, late pregnancy, anterior cruciate or meniscal tears, chondromalacia patellae.

THE POSE

1. Kneel with shins hip-width apart and parallel. Point your toes. Take a breath.
2. Do not close your throat or tighten stomach muscles as you reach behind to grasp your heels.
3. Transfer your weight backward by placing the heels of your hands on your heels as you advance your pelvis forward and arch your spine.
4. Slowly release your head backward. Make space by extending your hips.
5. Push upward with your heels into the palms of your hands. Use your hamstrings (not your quads) to elevate your pelvis. It will arch forward as your cervical spine arches back.
6. Inhale to raise your sternum as high as possible.
7. Here, too, breathe carefully. This time let the breath come from the front of the lower abdomen, and fill your lungs upward and backward, toward your shoulder blades, raising your entire chest upward toward the sky.
8. Exhale in the opposite order: from the back of the chest toward the front of the abdominal diaphragm.
9. Hold this pose from thirty seconds to one minute, breathing slowly and fully through your nose.

LESS CHALLENGING VARIATIONS

1. Kneel with the small of your back at the front of the seat of a chair, shins parallel beneath the chair. Point your toes. Place your hands on the seat of the chair, fingers pointing backward. Arch your back

against the front of the chair seat and gradually lower your head backward as you crawl your hands farther toward the back of the chair.

2. Kneel and sit back on a large pillow positioned on the backs of your
   parallel calves. Grasp your heels and gradually raise your pelvis forward and up, off the pillow.

Note: Often people will instinctively tighten their quadriceps while doing
Ustrasana, straightening their knees further and increasing the diameter of
the arch in this pose. However, the rectus femoris, one of the quadriceps,
crosses the groin and inserts on the pelvis. If it contracts, it reduces the angle
of the pelvis with the thigh and actually works against the total arching that
is the point of this pose. Relaxing the quadriceps and abdominal musculature
while contracting the hamstrings and gluteus maximus is much more effective, and yields a freer, more open, and greater arch, which is the goal here.

After you've done the pose, if you can, sit back down between your
heels, and walk your hands backward, away from your feet. Bend your
elbows in order to lower your lumbar spine to the mat (Supta Virasana).
Stretch your arms out over your head, parallel, palms up, elbows straight.
Elongate so the back of your head gets farther and farther away from the
shoulders on the mat. If you are not familiar with this pose, have a teacher
or friend help you lower your torso backward. Use pillows or a bolster if you
can't comfortably make it all the way to lying face up, with arms stretched
out against the mat.

FORWARD BENDS

Benefits and how they work: These poses compress the abdominal
organs, and thereby reduce impulses to eat, and also provide muscular balance,
since the backbends stretch the abdomen by contracting the dorsal region, and
these do the reverse. If you have spinal stenosis, these poses may help.

Contraindications: Herniated lumbar discs, hamstring tear, retrolisthesis.

Janu Sirsasana
Head-to-knee pose

Benefits and how it works: First, the name is misleading, since you
should not literally bring your head to your knees. Rather, the head comes

forward with a straight back. This tends to elongate the dorsal, or posterior, part of the digestive tract. The part of the stomach in the back, the fundus down to the pyloric antrum, is rich in the nerve fibers that transmit signals to the brain.

Contraindications: Herniated disc, hamstring tear, osteoporosis, coccygodynia, ischial bursitis.

Helpful hint: If you have difficulty bending from your hips, sit on one or two folded blankets.

THE POSE

1. Sit on a flat surface with your legs stretched out in front of you.
2. Bend your left knee, pressing the left foot high up on the right thigh. The right foot should be vertical.
3. Make your shoulders parallel to the two sides of your foot.
4. Tighten the right quadriceps, which will activate the agonist-antagonist reflex to relax the hamstrings and gluteal muscles.

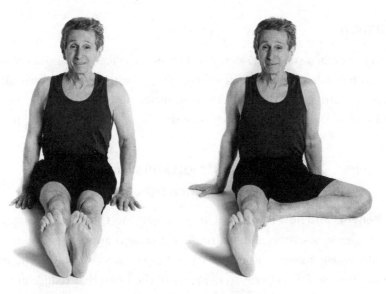

Janu Sirsasana,
head-to-knee pose—setup

Janu Sirsasana—
stage I

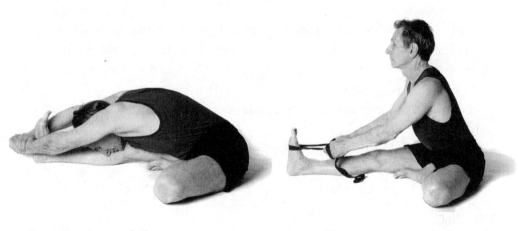

Janu Sirsasana—full pose   Janu Sirsasana—variation

5. With your back straight, bend your torso forward from your hips. Let your abdomen descend to your thigh, not your head to your knee. Advance your head forward toward your foot, not down toward your knee.
6. Grasp your left wrist with your right hand at your right foot's arch.
7. Breathe evenly and symmetrically in the position for thirty seconds to one minute. Then repeat with the legs reversed.

VARIATION

If you can't reach your toes, loop a belt around the foot of the straight leg. Pull with both hands equally, and crawl your fingers forward on the belt until your elbows are straight. Advance your head forward, toward the foot, not downward toward the knee, by pulling your shoulders back in a rowing motion.

Paschimottanasana
Extreme forward bend

Benefits and how it works: This pose helps in three ways. First, by pulling on the sciatic nerve, hamstrings, adductors, and gluteal muscles, and stimulating the many sensory nerves that are embedded within the muscles, it generates powerful signals to the parts of the brain that reduce anxiety and appetites of every kind. Second, through this same stretching, the forward-bending action slides the spinal cord a few millimeters downward within the spinal canal toward the legs. Mobilizing the spinal cord in this way also quiets the entire person. If you have spinal stenosis, this pose is beneficial, providing more room for the crowded nerve fibers within the spinal column.

Contraindications: Vertebral compression or other fracture, ostomies, ischial bursitis, herniated disc, osteoporosis, severe hip arthritis, total hip replacement (posterior approach).

Helpful hint: If you have difficulty folding from your hips, sit on a folded blanket.

THE POSE

1. Sit on a flat surface with your legs stretched out parallel to each other, inner ankles together.
2. Inhale and lengthen your spine.
3. Bend forward from your hips as you exhale. Grasp your feet, or catch one hand with the other beyond them, or hold a belt that goes across the soles of your feet above the arches and just below the ball of each foot.

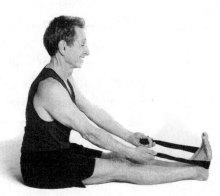

Paschimottanasana—with belt

4. Keep your ankles close together and toes brought up toward your knees (toes not pointed).
5. Reach forward, not down, resting your forehead and cheekbones and, if possible, your chin on the fronts of your legs.
6. Relax your elbows and the muscles between your legs; let the weight of your elbows pull you down. Breathe slowly and evenly to reduce any discomfort.

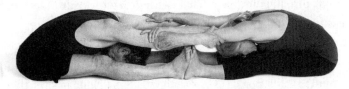

Paschimottanasana—for two

Ardha Baddha Padma Janusirsasana
Half lotus head-to-knee pose

Benefits and how it works: The bent leg's foot should fit under the rib cage, and the forward bending should therefore press against the abdomen, moving its contents backward and downward. This will produce some elongation of the entire duodenum and the stomach itself.

Posture: Tight hamstrings and lumbar muscular spasm are frequent companions of overweight; lower back pain and poor posture, such as hyperlordosis and kyphosis, quickly follow. This pose works against all that, conferring on the practitioner a pleasurable sense of a pliant lower back and lightness of leg. By stretching one leg at a time, the pose smoothly and naturally divides and conquers hamstring tightness and (in the bent leg) quadriceps tightness. The pressure of the lotus foot on the abdomen and the forward pull of the arms and abdominal muscles create agonist-antagonist reflexes that will calm and stretch the very tough quadratus lumborum muscles. A prime example of the agonist-antagonist reflex is in the arm: when the biceps bends the elbow, the triceps, which straightens the elbow, simultaneously relaxes. This reflex applies to each pair of muscles with opposite function: Contraction of one causes its opposite to loosen. This is called reciprocal inhibition, and it is useful in every version of this pose.

Contraindications: Osteoporosis, colostomy or recent abdominal surgery, concurrent herniated disc, severe knee or hip arthritis or replacement (posterior approach), sprained ankle, pregnancy.

Helpful hints: Use the straightest possible leg and place the lotus leg's foot as high up on the opposite thigh as you safely can. It is better to go forward farther with a slightly bent leg than to reduce the bend in order to keep the leg arrow-straight, even if it means sacrificing the reciprocal inhibition of the hamstrings and the quadriceps a little. But you'll get more stretch for the quadratus lumborum, in your lower back, with greater forward motion generating more pressure against the stomach itself, and therefore better inhibition of appetite. But if the leg is truly straight, inhibitory reflexes are activated that relax the hamstrings after thirty to sixty seconds.

Comment: In his book *Light on Yoga* B.K.S. Iyengar says that this pose "gives a good pull to the navel and abdominal organs."[4]

THE POSE

1. Sit with left leg stretched straight out, foot vertical. Face your shoulders toward the corners of your foot.
2. Inhale, then exhale as you bend your right knee and place the top of your right foot high up on the left thigh, your right heel against your mid-right lower abdomen.
3. Keeping your back straight, fold your torso forward.
4. Hold your left foot with both hands, or clasp your right wrist with your left hand beyond the foot. Coax your chest forward, not down. Exhale and relax your elbows. Let your elbows pull you forward as gravity draws them down.

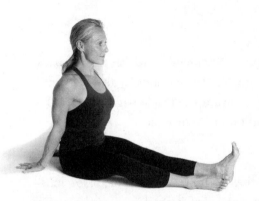

Ardha Baddha Padma Janusirsasana, half lotus forward bend—setup

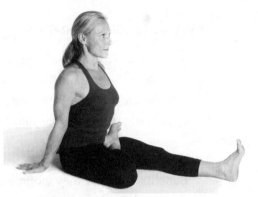

Ardha Baddha Padma Janusirsasana —first half

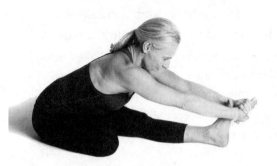

Ardha Baddha Padma Janusirsasana

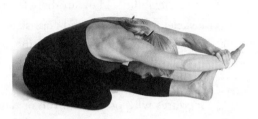

Ardha Baddha Padma Janusirsasana —intense

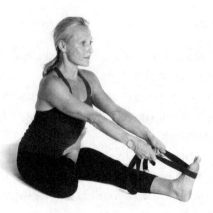

Ardha Baddha Padma Janusirsasana
—with belt

LESS CHALLENGING VARIATION

Loop a belt around the sole of your foot. Remember to keep your back straight. Creep your hands forward along the two strands of the belt until your elbows are straight. Aim your navel toward the inside (right side) of the left thigh, rather than aiming your head toward your knee.

TWISTING POSES

Benefits and how they work: Twisting pits one side of your torso's muscles against the other's. Your stomach is somewhat to the left of center; these poses rotate it back or forward, relative to your throat, depending on whether you're twisting to the left or right. In addition, the radial forces generated by twists are beneficial for strengthening vertebral bone, and, naturally, for truncal flexibility. They are beneficial for hip and mild facet arthritis, musculoskeletal back pain, and core strengthening as well.

Contraindications: Total hip replacement (posterior approach), herniated lumbar disc (best to twist away from the side of the herniation), vulnerability to shoulder subluxation, shoulder replacement, spinal fusion procedures with or without rod or wire, severe scoliosis, colostomy, ankylosing spondylitis.

Marichyasana III
Seated twist

Benefits and how it works: By twisting the neck, the rib cage and its contents (the lungs and great blood vessels), the stomach, and (to a lesser extent) the lumbar region, this pose stimulates the vagus nerve at multiple points. The vagus nerve, which is the longest nerve in the body, sends signals that travel all the way to the appetite centers in the brain; those centers have the ability to inhibit the desire to eat. The pose mechanically stretches the linings of the lungs, esophagus, stomach, and duodenum.

Contraindications: Vulnerability to subluxation/dislocation of the shoulder or of the hip (e.g., after shoulder or hip replacement, or due to severe arthritis); recently herniated disc; severe scoliosis; spinal fixation with Harrington rod, Cotrel-Dubousset, or fusion procedures; ankylosing spondylitis.

Helpful hints: Each time you breathe in, be aware of your posture, and remember to straighten your spine; each time you exhale, twist a little further. Use a blanket if needed to tip the pelvis forward. Avoid straining the muscles between your ribs, the intercostal muscles, by increasing the intensity of the pose gradually, and twisting from the lowest rib.

THE POSE

1. Sit with your legs extended straight forward. Sit on a folded blanket if needed to tip your pelvis forward.
2. Use your hands to pull your buttocks and upper thighs back and apart. Then use hand pressure on the mat to tip the pelvis forward properly.
3. Inhale to expand your chest, lifting the spine up powerfully. You can press your hands down on the floor beside you to get maximal lift.

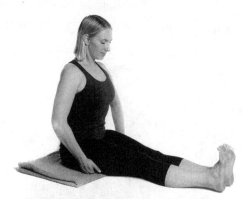

Marichyasana III, seated twist— preparing to twist

4. Bend your right knee and place the right foot flat on the mat on the medial (inside) or lateral (outside) of the left thigh.

5. Press the entire left leg down firmly, stretching fully through the sole of the foot. Especially stretch the big-toe side of the foot forward.

6. On your next inhalation, lift your spine again; on exhaling, turn toward the right.

7. Hook your left upper arm outside your right knee. Stretch the right arm straight.

8. Move the spine in and up with your inhalation and twist more with your exhalation. Lead the twist with your left lower ribs wrapping toward the right.

9. Turn your left arm inward to wrap it in front of and around your bent right leg, then reach toward your left thigh with the palm up.

10. Wrap your right arm behind your waist and clasp your hands, or use a belt to extend your reach.

11. With each inhalation, lift up and roll your right *shoulder* back. With each exhalation, press your left foot down and advance your left *chest* forward, twisting to the right.

12. Within the constriction of the pose, maintain a steady breath and a calm mind. Twisting poses teach focus and calm. Twisting to the right stretches the digestive tract. Twisting to the left conditions your digestive tract to be satisfied, enhancing your calm.

13. Rest for a moment, then repeat this on the other side.

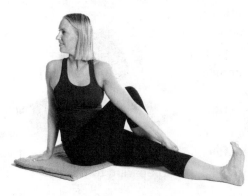

Marichyasana III—beginning twist

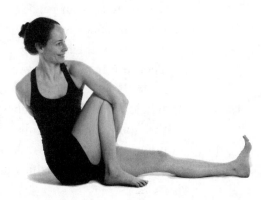

Marichyasana III—midway into twist

LESS CHALLENGING VARIATION 1

1. Sit on a folded blanket that does not extend below your thighs. That tilts your pelvis forward. Extend your legs straight out in front of you.
2. Use your hands to pull your buttocks and upper thighs back and apart to tip the pelvis even farther forward.
3. Inhale to expand your chest, lifting the spine up. Press your hands down on the floor beside you to lift the spine as much as possible.
4. Bend your right knee and place the foot on the mat lateral to (outside) the left thigh.
5. Anchor the left leg firmly down, stretching fully through the sole of the foot. Especially stretch the big-toe side of the foot forward.
6. On your next inhalation, lift your spine again and turn toward the right.
7. Place your left upper arm outside your right knee and raise your fore-arm to vertical. Press the outside of your knee with your elbow, and place your right hand on the floor for balance and to elevate your shoulders and straighten your spine.
8. Use the right elbow to draw the right shoulder back; walk your hand behind you to the left. Leverage the left elbow to draw the left chest forward.
9. Move the spine in and up with your inhalation, possibly elevating your chest more by raising your right hand up on its fingertips, while keep-ing the arm straight.

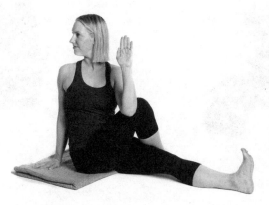

Marichyasana III (variation)— in progress

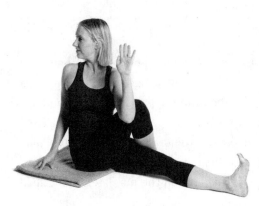

Marichyasana III

10. Twist more with your exhalation.
11. Breathe slowly and evenly, attempting to inflate both sides of the chest evenly in spite of their asymmetry in this pose.
12. Change legs and repeat on the opposite side.

LESS CHALLENGING VARIATION 2

1. Sit deeply in an armchair.
2. Place your left hand on the right arm of the chair.

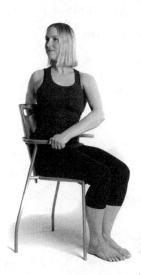

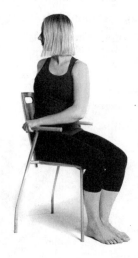

Marichyasana III—in chair setup   Marichyasana III—in chair full twist

3. Slide your right hand around behind the back of the chair toward the left arm of the chair. Take care to move your hips and knees as little as possible while you do this.

4. Now straighten up as you breathe in.

5. As you exhale, put gentle twisting pressure on your spine by gradually bending your elbows.

6. Then creep your hands toward each other in their respective directions, the left hand to the back of the right armrest, the right hand around the back of the chair to the left; straighten up again as you inhale, and reapply the twisting motion as you exhale.

7. Be careful not to round your back as you do this.

8. Repeat the "creep" two or three times, then hold the position, straightening your posture with each inhalation, and drawing the right shoulder back and pressing the left chest forward each time you exhale.

9. After one minute repeat on the other side.

Ardha Matsyendrasana I
Half Lord of the Fishes

Benefits and how it works: Bending the leg that was straight in Marichyasana III relaxes the hamstrings and puts slack in the iliotibial band, permitting further rotation and proportionately greater stimulus to the stretch receptors in the duodenum, stomach, and esophagus. If you have bone loss, this pose is beneficial.

Contraindications: Rotator cuff tear, herniated lumbar disc (best to twist to the opposite side), later pregnancy, severe scoliosis, ankylosing spondylitis, vertebral fixation by rods or wires, vertebral fracture, colostomy.

THE POSE

1. Sit on a folded blanket with your legs stretched out in front of you.

2. Manually widen your buttocks and thighs. This will help you to avoid a slumped posture. Your sit bones will move back. See page 83.

3. Bend your left knee and bring the foot outside your right hip, the knee on the floor pointing forward. Bend the right knee and place the right

foot flat on the floor to the outside of your left thigh, with the shin vertical. Place both hands on your right knee.

4. As you inhale, lift your spine up and simultaneously press down through the pelvic bones. Isometrically, though they will not move, attempt to widen your thighs. This will help your spine to lengthen for the twist.

5. As you exhale, asymmetrically contract your abdominal muscles, lengthen your tailbone down, and turn toward the right. Cross your left elbow to the outside of your right knee and point the hand and forearm upward.

6. Bring your right hand to the floor behind you and pause to breathe.

7. As you inhale, raise and straighten your spine; become taller. As you exhale, twist more, and walk your right hand around behind you toward the left.

8. Look over your right shoulder. Retain a vertically elongated spine and do not tilt your head.

9. Examine and equalize the downward pressure the pose exerts through both sides of the pelvis to stabilize the base of the pose.

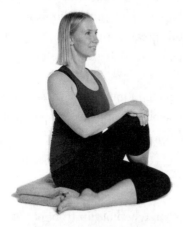

Ardha Matsyendrasana Half Lord of the Fishes— setup

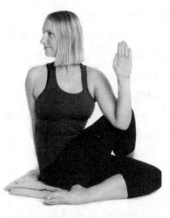

Ardha Matsyendrasana

10. Continue to breathe and soften internally to receive the twist. There may be a subtle inner turn still possible even when your spine and ribs appear to have reached their limits.

11. After several breaths, return to facing toward your right knee. Uncross your legs and stretch them straight in front of you.

12. Repeat all actions above on the other side.

13. After doing both sides, sit for a moment to feel the results of this pose, which does its work in many regions of the body.

Note: Lengthen the spine upward to free it and the rib cage for rotation. Press down through the pelvic bones. Use your abdominal muscles to help you twist.

Parivrtta Trikonasana
Twisted triangle

Benefits and how it works: Because so much twisting occurs between T12, the final vertebra to house a rib, and L1, the first lumbar segment, this is possibly the most effective pose in elongating and putting twist on the entire upper digestive tract, especially the gastroesophageal junction, where so many stretch receptors are located. For those with a "pain in the butt," piriformis syndrome, this pose beneficially stretches the piriformis muscle. Be sure to keep both your feet fully on the floor to prevent imbalances.

Note: One school of thought favors keeping the hips perpendicular to the plane of the legs and torso, and another encourages twisting the hips maximally and scissoring the thighs together. It is a question of whether to divide the twist into two parts and keep the sacroiliac joint out of it (perpendicular hips) or to make the entire body one large twist, thereby enabling the sacrum to do some of the twisting, which will take some of the pressure of the twist off the hips and lumbar spine. I believe you should endeavor to make one large full-body twist, from the back foot's heel to the nape of the neck. This will make for finer balance and will spread the twist evenly along the body, enabling one part to compensate for another and act as a "safety valve" if necessary. However, in sacroiliac joint derangement and following posterior-approach hip replacement, locking thighs at ninety degrees does have a point.

Contraindications: Second and third trimesters of pregnancy, herniated lumbar disc, acute sacroiliac joint derangement, severe spinal (facet) arthritis, colostomy.

THE POSE

1. Stand with feet three to three and a half feet apart, turn your right foot out ninety degrees, and turn your left foot thirty degrees inward.
2. Stretch your arms out horizontally, palms down.
3. Take a breath.
4. Exhale and twist to your right as you bend forward, pivoting your left hip forward until your left hand rests on the floor or on a block to the little-toe side of your right foot.
5. Scissor your legs together as you lengthen your spine.
6. Draw your shoulder blades together, aligning them as much as possible into the plane defined by the intersection of your legs.
7. Make your torso narrow and long.

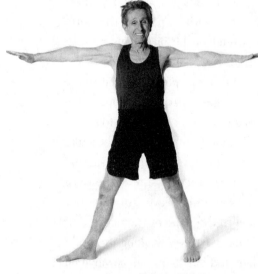

Parivrtta Trikonasana, Twisted Triangle—beginning

Parivrtta Trikonasana

VARIATION

1. Stand facing a wall with your left foot turned thirty degrees in toward the wall and close to it. Your right foot should be four inches away from the wall and parallel to it.
2. Stretch both arms out horizontally, palms facing downward.
3. Twist diagonally to the right, bending your left elbow as you first raise your arm above your head to clear the wall, and then descend toward the outside of your right foot.
4. Place your left palm on the floor with your little finger next to the right little toe. If you cannot reach that far, grasp your right ankle or calf with your left hand.
5. If it is difficult to reach down even that far, place your hand on a block or a chair.
6. Lean against the wall after you twist, reaching up and behind you with your right shoulder blade to place as much of your back as possible in contact with the wall.

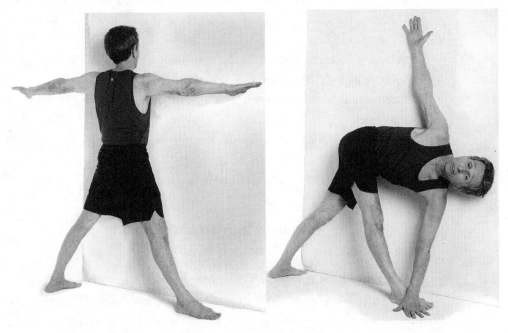

Parivrtta Trikonasana—at the wall

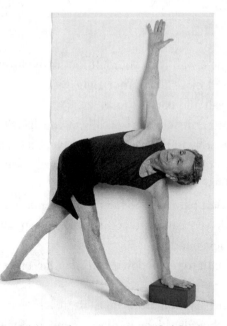

Parivrtta Trikonasana—with block

7. Using the wall and your left hand with its palm on the floor, your ankle, or the chair will help you work on the pose without worrying about your balance.
8. Scissor your legs together. Make your body as thin front to back and become as long, head to toe, as possible.
9. Stretch out; elongate from the backs of your thighs to the nape of your neck.
10. Hold the pose for thirty seconds. Breathe as slowly and symmetrically as possible.
11. Repeat on the other side, beginning by facing the wall.

Jathara Parivartanasana
Stomach twist

Benefits and how it works: This pose definitely stretches the gastro-intestinal tract through twisting. In addition, it coordinates the actions of the hips, sacroiliac joints, and lumbar spine, equalizing these three critical regions' participation in twists. That's why this posture goes some distance toward preventing the arthritis that comes from overtaxing one joint due to underutilizing another. It also reciprocally strengthens and stretches the external and internal oblique muscles and the transversus abdominis. In my experience, this pose has the extra benefit of giving relief in painful facet syndrome. Although there is no research confirming it at this writing, the pose also likely puts enough torque on lumbar vertebrae to improve bone mineral density.

Contraindications: Second and third trimesters of pregnancy, severe hip arthritis and recent hip replacement, trochanteric bursitis, colostomy, severe herniated lumbar disc, aortic aneurism, severe sacroiliac joint derangement.

THE POSE

1. Lie flat on your back.
2. Extend your arms out on the floor perpendicular to your body, palms up.
3. Take a breath and stretch your heels and your fingernail tips as far out from your torso as possible.
4. Exhale as you flex your knees and hips, both to ninety degrees.
5. Now straighten your knees so your legs are stiff as planks of wood.

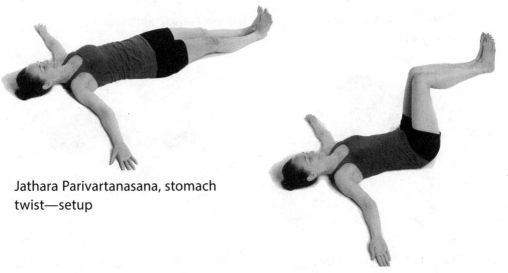

Jathara Parivartanasana, stomach twist—setup

Jathara Parivartanasana—starting

6. Tilt your buttocks off to the left.
7. Steadily lower your straightened legs to the right until your feet nearly touch your hands.
8. The left shoulder has a tendency to rise at this point. Press down with the back of the right hand and arm to bring your full back onto the mat.
9. Hold the pose for thirty seconds on each side.

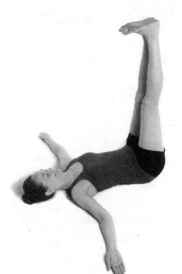

Jathara Parivartanasana—
halfway there

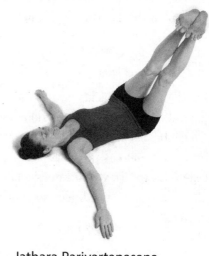

Jathara Parivartanasana—
in progress

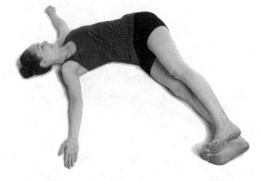

Jathara Parivartanasana

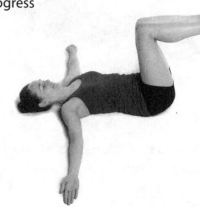

Jathara Parivartanasana (less challenging variation)—switching sides

LESS CHALLENGING VARIATION

1. Lie flat on your back.
2. Extend your arms out on the floor perpendicular to your body, palms up.
3. Take a breath and stretch your heels and the backs of your hands as far out from your torso as possible.
4. Exhale as you flex your hips and knees to ninety degrees.
5. Tilt your buttocks off to the left.
6. Now steadily lower your legs to the right until your knees nearly touch your forearms. If your heels don't come all the way down, refrain from using a block to support them.
7. Straighten your knees as much as you comfortably can. You can use your knees similar to a rheostat, initially keeping them bent to reduce strain, and straightening them little by little as you develop more strength, flexibility, and skill. This is analogous to the rheostat in a light switch with a sliding control that can smoothly raise or lower illumination.
8. The left shoulder has a tendency to rise at this point. Press down with the back of the right hand to bring your full back onto the mat.
9. Hold the pose for as close to thirty seconds as possible.
10. Repeat on the other side.

These are all the poses you need to begin to lose weight through yoga. Now we must turn to germane concerns about them and about yoga in general.

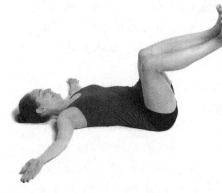

Jathara Parivartanasana—
using legs as a rheostat

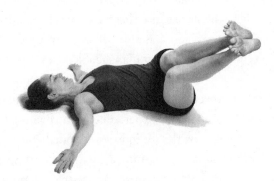

Jathara Parivartanasana—
turning up the rheostat

CHAPTER 8

Staying Safe to Gain the Benefits

HOW TO AVOID GETTING HURT

THOUGH YOUR GOAL is to use yoga to control your weight, it's worth paying attention to some other issues along the way, as they can impact your road to achievement. Sir Isaac Newton's first law implies that for every action, there is an equal and opposite reaction. Isn't it also reasonable that for everything that has an effect, there will be side effects? When it comes to the medications intended to reduce your weight, that seems to be an understatement, because there are five or ten adverse side effects to match each benefit. Yoga, too, has side effects, but they are few, almost invariably mild, and they are eminently manageable.

I did a study with Ellen Saltonstall and Susan Genis in which we surveyed 33,000 yoga teachers and students worldwide, asking nosy questions about their experience with yoga-related injuries.[1] First, there were the obvious truths: Standing on your head incorrectly can give you cervical pain or worse; going into a forward-bending pose too deeply and for too long can make your hamstring muscles ache the next day; and so on. However, the larger picture, the overall impression, was somewhat unexpected. There was almost unanimous agreement on the three biggest causes of injuries from all sources. Our conclusions were unexpectedly corroborated by a second, independent study, conducted in Australia.[2] According to both studies, the data from nearly 50,000 practitioners yield the three principal sources of yoga injuries.

TRYING TOO HARD

Whether from egotism, showing off, perfectionism, or an overenthusiastic embrace of yoga, the most common source of even slight injury is trying to do things that are currently beyond your capacity. Teachers desiring to be "role models" get themselves into trouble this way. Nevertheless, some surprising facts came out in both the Australian study and our own that actually make the point. On the same theme:

- Teachers are injured more than students: The desire to be the platonic ideal and the overarching impulse for perfection overcome common sense.
- More injuries occur in class than in at-home practice: This is the show-off/competitive impulse.
- Proportionally, men get injured more than women: A slight variation in the principle is operative in classes that are 80 percent young women: The men see the often more-flexible and adept women, then pit their stronger muscles against their poorer range of motion and, voilà, injuries occur.

Antidote: Pace yourself. Know your limits, and if you don't know them, stay a good distance on their estimated safe side. The analogy I like imagines a man walking on a desert, with a palm tree and a pyramid ahead in the distance, both framed by the horizon. As he walks farther, he will pass the palm tree, and then the pyramid. But he will never cross the horizon. Why not? Because he will be pushing the horizon farther off with each step. However, if he keeps on walking, he will definitely pass the place in the sand where the horizon was located when he started. That's the way it should be with your current limits and your goals in yoga. As you do yoga, first you can seek immediate, easy-to-reach objectives; then the larger, more perfectionistic goals will definitely be attainable, but they will take time. After a while you will be able to do things that, if tried at first, would have injured you. But there will still be limitations, so keep common sense at the forefront.

POOR ALIGNMENT

What is alignment? Fundamentally, it is conforming to the natural curves and essential leeways in the spine, and the joints of the appendages, especially the shoulders, hips, and knees. Of course poor alignment can be exacerbated by overweight, just as it can come "naturally" to those who just want to lose two pounds. No matter what they weigh, many people are just misinformed about what their muscles and joints *can* do, and even more are in the dark about what their muscles and joints *should* be doing. Anatomical ignorance is rampant. After a discussion with a colleague about this, we asked all the people in a beginner yoga class to show us where their livers were. Half the group put their hands on their left sides. They needed education and body awareness, two things practicing yoga promotes.

As sole proprietors of our bodily actions, we have a very good idea of our physical limitations by the time we reach our teens. Desiring to go beyond our limits, either seeking perfection or through exaggerated enthusiasm, competitiveness, or just plain showing off, we sometimes go ahead and do things we should know better than to try. In the yoga I am showing you, the advice about what you should do will always be a subset of what you can do. Only you intimately know your physical abilities and limitations.

Proper yoga estimates the tolerable forces that may be applied to the joints of your shoulders, hips, and knees and offers poses within these bounds. So, for example, in Virabhadrasana I, the Warrior I, the forward thigh, shin, and foot are all in the same plane. Otherwise, skewed forces will endanger the hip and ankle, and especially the unsecured knee. Please remember, I offer safer and gentler ways to begin doing poses, and common mistakes to guard against. There's truth in the old saw: When in doubt, don't.

INADEQUATE TEACHING

This is the third-most-common cause of yoga injury. How do you pick the right class? The rule I follow is: one teacher or alert assistant for every fifteen students or, better yet, each ten. Inattention to new students is probably the most egregious error for any teacher, where initial false steps may be dangerous, and bad practices are always harder to correct later. In yoga this may be particularly true, where false steps may become harmful when repeated many times. Size of class versus number of staff is something any beginner can easily calculate and use as a guide.

But there are other aspects of teaching that have an influence on injury. I consider five years of teaching desirable for any teacher who has a new student with a special condition, including overweight. That is enough time for a teacher to have seen the common problems and know how to deal with them, at least with regard to safety. The teacher should ask you about your medical history, and also ask about your goals in yoga. The room should be clean, light, and big enough for the students to stretch out and feel they are on their own.

Then come the less tangible aspects of the teacher-student relationship: Do you have respect for the teacher, and trust and feel comfortable with what you are encouraged to do? Do you like her or him? Making up your mind about these things may take a few sessions, or more, but do not be timid about changing after any amount of time: You can injure your body, but even more serious, you can also damage your enthusiasm. You don't want—under any circumstances—to divert yourself from your goal.

INCIDENTAL SUCCESS

Adrienne was a 5'3" college sophomore weighing 179 pounds when she happened to read a brochure about a free yoga class. She had heard of yoga, was mildly curious, and since the price was right and finals were over, she bought herself a roomy pair of shorts, a loose top, and took them with her to the studio, still in the bag from the store. The ninety-minute class tired her out, but she really liked it, and she signed up for ten lessons before she left. Registering for the next semester, she noticed she was fitting in her classes around her yoga, even though she could have changed the yoga lessons' times, and she'd only had one class so far. Fortunately, she got all her requisite courses and still allotted enough time to get to and from the yoga classes. "I didn't even notice it. The girl sitting next to me in American History told me she thought I was thinner than I was before. I weighed myself and I'd gone from 179 to 165. That was in the third week of the term."

Adrienne was a good student, and a good yoga student too. She kept the twice-a-week yoga schedule and started doing about twenty minutes of yoga a day in her room. Heading into Easter she weighed herself again: 152. "I took my yoga mat home to Michigan over spring break," she says.

> I wasn't thinking so much about losing weight, honestly. I just thought I'd miss the yoga so much. Though there were many yoga studios in Grand Rapids, I'd never noticed; I didn't go to any of the local places. It felt good to do the program that I'd learned at home for about forty-five minutes twice a day. What amazed me was that the food my folks made for lunch and for dinner didn't interest me the same way, and I didn't eat as much.
>
> I thought that by doing yoga before meals I'd probably work up a bigger appetite. It turned out to be just the reverse. I was leaving things on my plate, something my mother said she'd never seen me do before . . . never. By the time I returned to school for finals, my weight was down in the 140s, and I was looking at three As and a B-plus. In a little over four months I'd lost close to forty pounds and improved my grade-point without really trying to do either! No exercise schedule has ever held me for more than a couple of weeks. I guess I really just liked doing yoga.

Now, sixteen years later, Adrienne is working part-time at a midwestern law firm. In spite of giving birth to two children and attending a good many office parties, she weighs 124. She still does yoga daily, as do her nine- and five-year-olds.

Adrienne's story is hardly unique. It illustrates how yoga can alter your appetite and your mindset, more than anything else, even without your intention to do so. Possibly she also improved her self-discipline, which could account for her better grades, but that was not involved in the weight loss. Mitochondria could obviously figure in here. Initially she had no interest in any of these things; it was something the yoga did without any conscious help from her.

But we do not all have Adrienne's temperament. She took up yoga on a whim, but when she found out what it was, she stuck to it, and has for many years. For some, setting a goal is a critical part of sticking to any program or project. Most people will find that yoga is the sort of thing that helps you keep your promise to yourself, and does improve your willpower, or self-discipline, or whatever you choose to call it. Yoga will also help you refine your goal. It can alter your appetite, what you eat and how much you eat, but that is not all. Yoga can and very often does change a person's attitude—both your approach to other people and your perception of self.

Yoga "insidiously" turns your mind and bodily systems away from ingestion and digestion as the chief acts in your life. You end up spending more time thinking about whether what you're doing makes sense: Was it rational, was it generous, was it kind, or was it totally selfish? Yoga changes your outlook, the way it changed Adrienne's, who told me yoga gave her more respect for herself and for everything.

To many writers throughout the past two thousand years, yoga has been considered a bona fide and unlocked gateway to wisdom: There is a clear belief that yoga will improve not just your lifestyle, and the length of your life, but the quality of your experience in the life you lead. This will occur in ways you can perceive, like your weight, but in other ways that just happen, like the mitochondria and telomeres busily at work in your body without your awareness or consent.

CHAPTER 9

How to Design and Use Pose Sequences

We HAVE OUTLINED and described twelve poses that contribute to weight control. What is the best way to use them to accomplish your goal? Being practical, ask yourself: Which poses can you use, and when can you use them? In our complex and innovative lives, we may find ourselves in a great variety of circumstances fifteen to thirty minutes before mealtime.

STANDING SEQUENCES

Out at a meeting, at a sporting event, on public transportation, in many types of work, and in many other circumstances, there's nowhere to sit or lie down and do yoga. Sometimes only standing poses are possible, and then only for short periods. Those I have described in detail in the last chapter—Tadasana, the Mountain; Vriksasana, the Tree; Virabhadrasana I, the Warrior I; and Parivrtta Trikonasana, the Twisted Triangle (not with pregnancy)—are perfect for this type of situation. Tadasana is a unitary pose, and the other three have right-sided and left-sided versions. Together they are seven different positions. If each is held for one full minute, that's seven minutes in all.

SITTING SEQUENCES

Doing the sitting poses and the sitting twists is necessary when riding in an automobile or an airplane or a train; being anyplace with a low ceiling; or having knee or ankle pain, spinal stenosis, plantar fasciitis, spinal compression fracture, or a balance problem. Fortunately Ustrasana, the Camel; Marichyasana III, the seated twist (not with pregnancy); and Ardha Matsyendrasana, Half Lord of the Fishes (not with pregnancy) fit these conditions very well. It may seem a little daunting to kneel in the back seat of the car or twist in your chair before you finish writing a memo, but these actions will help you avoid a craving for french fries at lunch.

There are the myriad people with back disorders, something that overweight makes significantly more probable and more painful. People with spinal stenosis will gravitate toward the forward-bend sequence of Janu Sirsasana, Paschimottanasana, and Ardha Baddha Padma Janusirsasana (none of these have good English translations, so take a look at the pictures and descriptions in chapter 7). Herniated disc sufferers will benefit most from the back-bending Salabhasana, the Locust; Salabhasana, the Bridge; and Ustrasana, the Camel. Those with cauda equina syndrome, facet syndrome, or spinal stenosis may find some relief doing forward bends.

APPETITE-REDUCING SEQUENCES

While there is a general rule about delaying eating before yoga, there are also sequences of poses that will be beneficial. Doing a number of poses in a certain order can help bring about a decrease in appetite. Depending on the circumstances and your goals, the most sensible and effective sequences will feature variety in their structure.

Take, for example, Tadasana (page 63), Salabhasana (page 69), Janu Sirsasana (page 76), and Marichyasana (page 20). Tadasana, establishes good posture and a secure and solid calm. Salabhasana augments an energetic alertness and strengthens muscle groups that will improve posture, refine the mechanics of breathing, and simultaneously inhibit appetite by activating the stretch receptors in the gastrointestinal tract. Janu Sirsasana stretches the very anatomy that was strengthened through contraction in Salabhasana, and also stimulates the stretch receptors in the stomach, esophagus, and duodenum. Marichyasana helps define the abdomen as distinct from the chest, stimulates all three sections of the gastrointestinal tract to reduce appetite, and prompts relaxation in the legs, the back, the thorax, and even the face, retempering the heightened state invoked by Salabhasana. The four poses, done in that order, are a self-contained experience that should leave you more alert, but calmer and not as hungry as you were when you started.

Even these few poses give good combinations that will achieve what you want. Still, one must stave off the aura of boredom that can hover over and erode your intention to do repetitive daily exercise of any kind. We can construct good sequences for day-to-day variety, giving effective appetite control and self-awareness. Try these at first. After a while you may be able to make up your own.

Balanced Set

Vriksasana (Tree, page 64)

Setu Bandhasana (Bridge, page 71)

Paschimottanasana (Extreme Forward Bend, page 78)

Marichyasana (Straight-Leg Twist, page 83)

Invigorating Set

Virabhadrasana I (Warrior I, page 67)

Ardha Baddha Padma Janusirsasana (Half-Bound Lotus, page 80)

Salabhasana (Locust, page 69)

Ardha Matsyendrasana I (Bent-Knee Twist, page 87)

Quiet Set

Tadasana (Mountain, page 63)

Ustrasana (Camel, page 73)

Janu Sirsasana (Head-to-Knee, page 76)

Parivrtta Trikonasana (Twisted Triangle, page 89)

Mixed Set

Vriksasana (Tree, page 64)

Virabhadrasana I (Warrior I, page 67)

Ardha Matsyendrasana I (Bent-Knee Twist, page 87)

Paschimottanasana (Extreme Forward Bend, page 78)

These four different sequences can be rotated day by day, so three are done every day—one before breakfast, one before lunch, and one before dinner. Since there are four sets, it won't have to be the same order every day of the week for four weeks, or it can be more varied, depending on your work situation, traveling circumstances, and many, many other things. These sequences can also be used to govern, augment, or modify your mood.

If it is daunting to start something as new and different as yoga can be to the uninitiated, then start doing yoga before one meal a day. It makes sense to approach the biggest or most caloric meal: Do one of these sets fifteen to thirty minutes before that meal every day for a few weeks. First, that should give you a feel for what you are undertaking, and second, it will begin to dawn on you how spiritual it really is to be alive, with your physical frame like a sacred object. You will almost certainly have a better sense of how dramatically eating changes the way you feel, the way you perceive your entire body, and your efforts to do almost anything. It's likely that you will begin to shed some pounds.

Although yoga and overweight are very generally at opposite ends of the physical-fitness spectrum, a number of excellent and versatile yoga practitioners who may be just one size larger than they would like to be are interested in getting thinner. For them I have assembled a short set of "extra credit" asana that experienced yogis may want to tackle before meals.

"EXTRA CREDIT" POSES FOR EXPERIENCED YOGIS

Yoga and overweight are usually eminently separable, but there are some individuals who have practiced regularly for years and are heavy. They will have done most or all of the poses we've given, and some may even have intentionally done them fifteen to thirty minutes before meals. For them the above poses may not be enough, and so here are some more suggestions. These are all difficult postures; some poses may be new even to veteran yoga practitioners. Please read over the entire section on each pose before trying it. The "beginner" version is given after instructions for the classical pose. This way even first-timers in a pose will have a good idea where they are headed.

Sirsasana
The headstand

I have met a fair number of people who are excellent yoga practitioners yet never have even tried the headstand. There is a fear of it that seems to be based on reports of injuries. I believe these injuries have occurred because the pose was done incorrectly. I have been standing on my head for half an hour for decades without any injury, and many Iyengar colleagues have similar histories. It is a shame to miss this pose, called "the king of asana." These simple instructions should suffice, but if doubts linger, find an experienced teacher for the first few times you try.

Benefits and how it works: At the back of his classic text *Light on Yoga*, B.K.S. Iyengar has an index of many medical conditions and the asana that are best for relieving their unpleasant symptoms.[1] Fully three-quarters of these lists of beneficial asana begin with Sirsasana, the headstand. Yet in the Western world, with its fears and larger and possibly more litigious yoga classes, along with cervical injuries, glaucoma, and cerebrovascular conditions, the headstand is frequently neglected.

Still, if the contraindications do not apply to you, there is next to nothing that will give you a clearer and stronger sense of your body, an introduction to your own versatility, a novel "point of view," and a reprogramming of your gastrointestinal and vascular dynamics.

When you are inverted, every time you inhale, your diaphragm is virtually doing weight lifting with much of the weight of your stomach and intestines. This strengthens that life-giving muscle and simultaneously prompts you to develop greater breath control.

Contraindications: Glaucoma (wide- or narrow-angle), cervical disc disease, fracture, muscular imbalance, cerebrovascular accident (stroke), cerebrovascular disease, cerebral or carotid aneurism, epidural or subdural hematoma, severe congestive heart failure, arrhythmias, Wolff-Parkinson-White syndrome, severe hyper- or hypotension, glenohumoral (shoulder) dislocation, Sprengel's deformity, Klippel-Feil syndrome, Arnold-Chiari malformation, moderate or severe imbalance.*

---

* For a definitive list of contraindications, see www.YIP.guru.

Helpful hints: Use the center of your head. Do not balance on your forehead or the back of your skull; these alternative balance points are dangerous. Most of the weight should rest upon the crown of your head, the fontanelles. Your position inevitably changes from time to time; even long-standing yoga practitioners must frequently adjust the position of their arms and the angle of their heads during Sirsasana. It is important to do this and avoid the upside-down versions of "swayback," lordosis, and kyphosis.

Encouragement for beginners: Many yoga classes and even teacher-training programs totally avoid the "king of poses" for a variety of reasons. In my experience and that of like-minded colleagues, the headstand, properly done, is only very rarely involved in injuries of any kind.

THE POSE

1. Place a folded blanket in the middle of a room.
2. Interlock your fingers completely, bringing the heels of your hands together.
3. Kneel down and form an equilateral triangle in the middle of the blanket with your forearms.
4. Place the fontanelles, the crown of your head, where there was a soft spot when you were an infant, in the center of the triangle. Your wrists should contact the back of your head.
5. Retain symmetry as you increase the pressure on your forearms by walking in toward your eyes with your toes. Take care not to spread the elbows farther apart.

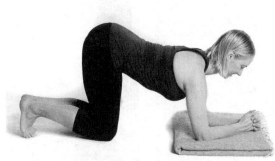

Sirsasana, the headstand—setup

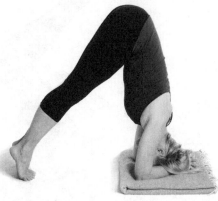

Sirsasana—first moves

6. As your torso approaches vertical, smoothly lift your feet from the floor. At first your knees may be bent, but with practice you'll be able to do this with completely straight legs.

7. Manage flexion and extension at the hips to retain vertical legs. Your ankles, hips, shoulders, and ears should be in one plane.

8. Raise your shoulders away from the floor; widen them, away from your ears. Keep your elbows where they are.

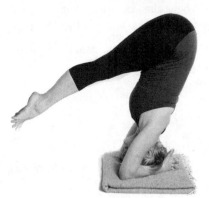

Sirsasana—lift off

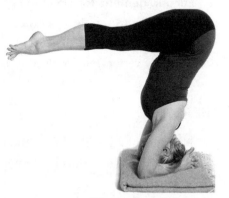

Sirsasana—legs rising

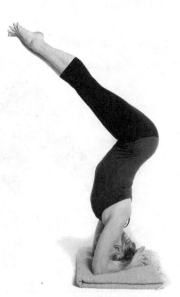

Sirsasana—nearing completion

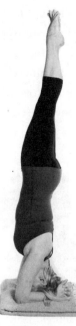

Sirsasana

9. Again equalize the pressure on your two forearms and between each elbow and each wrist.

10. Gradually work up to five and a half minutes in the pose.

11. Reverse the steps outlined above to come down from the headstand. At first bend your knees, but land on your toes.

12. It is preferable to go up and come down with both legs together, but that may be difficult at first.

EASIER ALTERNATIVE FOR BEGINNERS

(*Note:* This pose should be done with a friend who will stand behind you, spot you, and prevent you from falling over backward.)

1. Sit on a blanket facing a wall with legs straight out in front of you and feet in comfortable contact with the wall.

2. Mark the spot where you are sitting.

3. Turn over and kneel, facing down at the place you have marked.

4. Interlock your fingers and bring the heels of your hands together.

5. Place the little-finger sides of the hands on the blanket, forming an equilateral triangle, and place the crown of your head in the center of the triangle, on the marked spot, facing the wall.

6. Extend your legs to the wall and walk up the wall with your feet until they are just above horizontal. Your torso should come close to vertical.

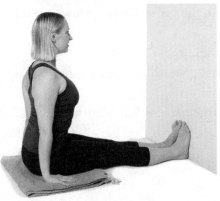
Sirsasana (easier alternative)—
marking the spot

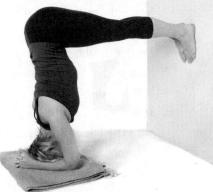
Sirsasana (easier alternative)—
Rising with assistance of wall

7. Stay in this position for half a minute at first, and longer thereafter.

8. Come down by walking down the wall. Take care that your toes reach the floor first, not your knees.

9. If you should fall backward, release your hands and bend your knees, letting your body go limp and flexible. Falling backward is not nearly as bad as it sounds.

After practicing for a while, when you feel secure and stable in the posture, invite a friend to help you balance and place the blanket in the corner of a room, as per the below.

Second, more challenging beginner version: Use the corner of a room, such that the outer ankles or heels are in contact with the perpendicular walls when you are inverted. Practicing against a single wall tends to make the legs arch back and the abdomen protrude forward. That can cause pain in the back and the neck, and it is stressful to the sense organs lodged in the head.

1. Place a folded blanket in the corner of a room.

2. Kneel with the outer corner of the folded blanket pointing between your legs.

3. Follow the directions for full headstand, possibly getting a friend to help you bring your legs over your head at first.

4. Let your feet or ankles or heels contact the two walls of the corner.

5. One by one, gradually advance your feet toward the center and slightly forward until neither is in touch with the walls. This may take several sessions or more.

6. Retreat to the walls if instability arises.

7. Stay up for half a minute at first, and gradually increase to five and a half minutes.

8. If you can, carefully follow the instructions for full headstand above, with the friend spotting you. If you are unstable, go back to the corner of a room for a week or two longer.

Parivrtta Parsvakonasana
Revolved side-angle pose

Benefits and how it works: This is about as twisty as a pose can get. The leverage on your entire torso is generated by powerful opposition between the shin of one leg firmly planted on the floor and the forearm of the opposite arm doing its best to revolve your torso. Any part of the digestive tract that is not tethered will be exposed to maximal torque. Being in the middle of this body torque, maximal stretch is applied to the esophagus, stomach, and duodenum.

This pose also coordinates a stretched piriformis muscle with major muscle groups above and below it, so it is excellent if you have the form of sciatica called piriformis syndrome.

By applying a great deal of torque to the vertebral bodies, and putting the forward and back hips under different but equal pressure, this pose stimulates bone deposition and could be one of the group of twelve poses that reverse osteoporosis.[2]

Contraindications: (Absolute): pregnancy; (Relative): poor balance, herniated disc, most types of hernia, history of spinal surgery, anterior shoulder subluxation/dislocation, severe knee or hip arthritis, total hip replacement (posterior approach), anterior cruciate or medial meniscal tear, colostomy.

THE POSE

1. Stand with feet four and a half to five feet apart.
2. Turn your right foot out ninety degrees and your left foot inward thirty degrees.
3. Retaining a vertical torso, bend your right knee to ninety degrees so the right shin is vertical and the thigh is horizontal.
4. Distribute the weight evenly over the four corners of your right foot.
5. In a coordinated movement thrust your left hip, chest, and shoulder forward and to the right, curling the outer left armpit around the outside of the right knee.
6. Place your left palm beside your right foot, while extending your right arm diagonally behind your ear and above your head.

7. Form a single diagonal line including your left leg, your right arm, and the upper border of your twisted torso.

8. Stretch from the outer edge of your left foot and your heel to your right fingertips, and pull back against the mat with your left hand to restrain your right chest from bulging upward.

9. Breathe symmetrically and smoothly.

10. Hold the pose for as close to thirty seconds as possible.

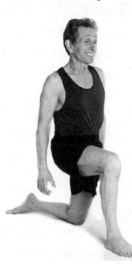

Parivrtta Parsvakonasana, revolved side-angle pose—setup

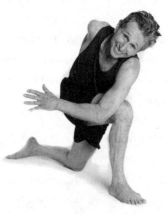

Parivrtta Parsvakonasana— beginning to twist

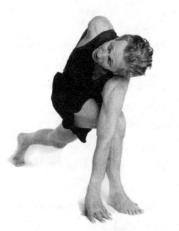

Parivrtta Parsvakonasana— further twist

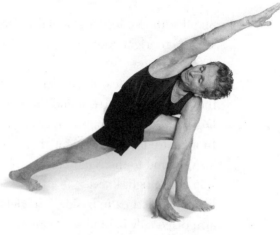

Parivrtta Parsvakonasana

LESS CHALLENGING VARIATION

1. Stand with feet four and a half to five feet apart with a wall several inches behind you.
2. Turn your left foot out so it is parallel to the wall; turn your right foot inward thirty degrees.
3. Retaining a vertical torso, bend your left knee to ninety degrees so the left shin is vertical and the thigh is horizontal.
4. Distribute half your weight equally among the four corners of your left foot. The other half is, of course, on your right foot.
5. Bend your right knee so you are kneeling on the mat.
6. In a coordinated movement thrust your right hip, chest, and shoulder forward and to the left, placing your right and left hands on the wall, and your right elbow just beyond the left knee and in contact with the outside of the left thigh.
7. Use your right hand to balance, twist, and maintain your left shin in a vertical position, and your left hand against the wall to balance and get more twist.

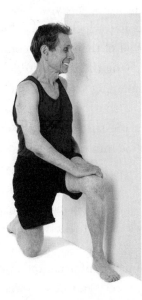

Parivrtta Parsvakonasana—
training version

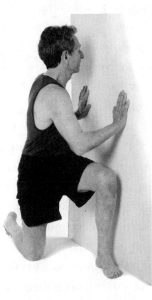

Parivrtta Parsvakonasana—
intermediate training version

8. Twist at the lowest waist, and between the ribs and the lumbar spine, not just at the shoulders.
9. With substantial contact between your right elbow and your left thigh, pull the elbow (without actually moving it) toward your upper thigh and torso to keep the chest from puffing out upward (not pictured).
10. Breathe evenly and calmly.
11. Stay in the pose for thirty seconds.

Urdhva Dhanurasana
The Wheel

Benefits and how it works: By producing an extreme arch, this very challenging pose stretches the gastrointestinal tract just about maximally, so much so that you likely stretch even the biliary tract, the tube running from the liver to the gall bladder, which, further down along its course, joins a tube from the pancreas. The bladder, ureters, and urethra get elongated; the ovaries and fallopian tubes do too. If anything is going to inhibit your appetite, stretching from your larynx to your ankles is likely the thing to do it.

Elongating and arching the back as this pose so brazenly does imitates the key move in McKenzie-type physical therapy, which is good for herniated disc, producing a partial vacuum at the front of the intervertebral spaces between the vertebral bodies, and thereby drawing the disc material toward its proper location, away from nerve roots emerging from the back of the spinal column.

The mammoth arch of the pose puts great pressure on the posterior elements of the spine, stimulating them to add bone mineral density, for anyone who has osteopenia or osteoporosis.

Last, it is almost impossible to maintain a depressed outlook in this exhilarating pose. Although no "permanent" changes in mood can ever be guaranteed, a relief, however temporary, gives a lightness and hope, even when you feel dismal.

Contraindications: (Absolute): Arnold-Chiari malformation; (Relative): sacroiliac joint derangement, spinal stenosis, facet syndrome, anterolisthesis, spondylolysis, Klippel-Feil syndrome, Sprengel's deformity, cerebrovascular disease.

THE POSE

1. Lie on your back on a sticky mat.
2. Bend your knees, placing your feet hip-width apart and parallel.
3. Dig your hands into the mat, palms down, under your shoulders, fingers angled slightly outward.
4. Strongly retract your shoulders downward toward your pelvis as you pull your arm bones toward their shoulder joints, and begin to press your palms down into the mat.
5. Inhale deeply as you lengthen your spine, elevate your pelvis, and lift your shoulders off the mat, putting a subtle head-to-toe arch into your back ribs.
6. Regain your balance and orientation in this position, with only your head and hands and feet on the mat.
7. Attend to the four corners of both feet.
8. Apply enough force on the mat with your hands to lift your chest high enough to place the top of your head on the mat.
9. Take a slow, easy breath.

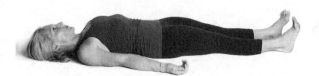

Urdhva Dhanurasana, the Wheel—
initial position

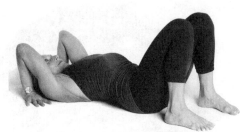

Urdhva Dhanurasana—beginning

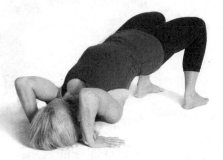

Urdhva Dhanurasana—
beginning ascent

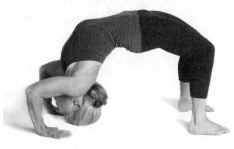

Urdhva Dhanurasana—halfway there

10. After exhaling, time your inhalation to your ascent, reaching a full breath as your elbows straighten completely.
11. Feet and palms on the floor, pause again for another full, slow breath.
12. Now, without moving your feet, press them against the mat and in the direction away from your head and torso. This will elevate and advance your chest, bringing your sternum more over your chin, and your shoulders directly above your hands.
13. At maximum elevation, armpits hollow, shoulder blades and back ribs impelling your chest forward, head suspended from the bridge of your spine, take a few slow, satisfying breaths.
14. Descend slowly by releasing the backward pressure on your feet, and the downward push of the hands and elbows, and the backward thrust of the shoulders. All this occurs as you slowly bend your elbows. Focus to make this a coordinated effort.
15. Let the back of your head rest on the mat for a few breaths before going on.

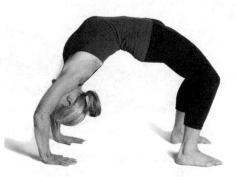

Urdhva Dhanurasana—further
elevating by straightening elbows

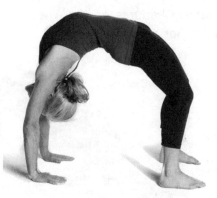

Urdhva Dhanurasana

Krounchasana
Heron Pose (easier than the Wheel, above)

Benefits and how it works: Like more sedate forward bends, this difficult pose will compress abdominal contents. Unlike most others, it will also forcibly activate abdominal and back muscles to work in a coordinated synchrony, since front-to-back balance is critical to the pose. The pose is exhilarating, and brings your thinking, your mood, and, in my experience, even your metabolism away from a focus on food.

Like Trianga Mukhaikapada Paschimottanasana, this pose emphasizes the alternate and reciprocal actions of the ankles. This is beneficial for those with plantar fasciitis because it reverses the pathological co-contraction of ankle flexors and extensors, which is the main cause of fascia-tearing forces on the arches of the feet.

Contraindications: (Absolute): posterior hip replacement; (Relative): abdominal or inguinal hernia, severe osteoporosis, severe or recent herniated disc, knee pathology such as meniscal or cruciate ligamentous tears, extreme knee or hip arthritis or knee replacement, sprained ankle.

Helpful hints: Manually pull the bent leg's calf muscles to the sides to enable you to sit on both ischial bones. Keep your back straight. Bring your leg to your forehead, not vice versa.

THE POSE

1. Bend your left knee beneath you and sit to the inside of your left calf, right leg stretched straight out before you. You will naturally list to the right. Correct this by equalizing the weight on your sit bones. Place a block or blanket under the right buttock if necessary.

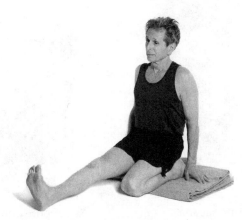

Krounchasana, the Heron—setup

2. Bend your right knee and lift it. Hold your right foot with both hands, or clasp your left wrist with your right hand around it.
3. Exhale as you straighten and raise your right leg to your forehead or, better, your chin.
4. Use your arms to raise your head up in line with your vertical leg and toward your foot.
5. Rise up further with each exhalation for thirty seconds of smooth breathing.
6. Inhale again as you slowly lower the right leg.
7. Repeat on the other side.

LESS CHALLENGING VARIATIONS

1. Balance can be an issue in this pose. If so, sit with your heel to a wall for front-to-back stability, and place both hands on the mat to keep yourself from falling to the back.
2. Loop a belt just behind the ball of the straight or almost-straight leg. Hold the belt as you raise the leg toward vertical. As you do this, place the other hand on the floor or on a block beside the foot of the bent leg.

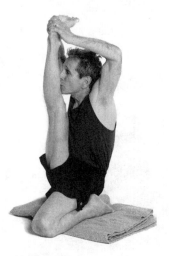

Krounchasana

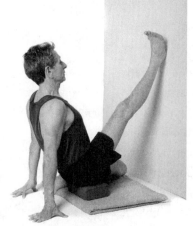

Krounchasana—
easier version

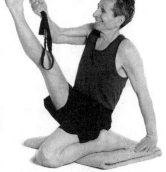

Krounchasana—
further adaptation for
balance and stiffness

KNOWING WHEN TO SAY WHEN

My cousin Martha visited us for a week at a summer house we had rented on a lake in Connecticut. Every afternoon she complained that her feet hurt. Some nights she would not even venture out with us as we strolled on the soft sand of the beach. She was an excellent educational administrator and a gifted clinical psychologist. She was 5'1" tall and weighed 160 pounds.

I dutifully examined her feet, and found nothing puzzling enough even to merit an X-ray. Those feet were fine.

"What could it be?" she inquired, her face and manner mild and receptive.

I responded without even thinking. "You know," I began, "when your arms and your midsection and your legs get big, your feet don't change. They stay pretty much the same."

Martha looked down and had to admit it. "Pretty much."

"When everything else expands, the feet don't."

"Right."

"So you have the same surface area bearing more and more pressure."

"True."

"Have you ever gone hiking with a backpack?"

"I used to love that."

"Did you stop because your feet hurt?"

"Actually, I think so."

"Well, now you have a built-in backpack."

Martha, age forty-nine, looked up with concerned astonishment and asked, "So what can I do? Those horrible pills? I hate boring exercises. Your wife's a wonderful cook. Listen, I'm on vacation!"

I described to her a way that she could eat whatever she wanted, just about as much as she wanted, anytime she wanted to, and all she had to do was quit eating a little early—a little before she normally finished. I told her that the stomach, like the bladder, is smooth muscle, the kind of muscle that expands to house just about anything you put in it. And if you leave the table just 5 percent hungry, for just a week or so, the stomach will start to contract.

"So I'll just be hungry for a week," Martha zipped back in joking sarcasm.

"More like an hour," I replied. "Remember when you were a kid, and we weren't allowed to eat cookies after four o'clock?"

"They said if we did, we wouldn't be able to eat our dinners at five thirty?"

"Yes, but why? Because the cookies went into our stomachs, quickly got digested into glucose, went into and circulated through the bloodstream, and turned off the appetite centers in our young brains. The same thing happens if you leave the table a little hungry at seven thirty."

"Dinner gets digested and pretty soon turns off the appetite centers in our adult brains?" she said, beginning to understand what I was getting at.

"So by nine o'clock, even though you left the table a little hungry, and haven't eaten anything since seven thirty, magically you're not hungry at all."

"And I'm only 5 percent hungry before that!"

Martha liked the idea, and lost about a pound a week for months. By April she weighed around 140. When she came to visit the next summer, it was like one of those before-and-after infomercials. She looked healthy, fit, happy, and, all in all, just right.

When I can, I use yoga in my practice of medicine. Though the method I used for my cousin isn't exactly yoga, it really seemed to help. I have also tried this same method for patients with herniated discs or dislocated sacroiliac joints, the patients for whom weight seemed to be a decisive factor in—the cause of—their back pain. It has worked apparent miracles for many.

SLEEPING TOO LITTLE, EATING TOO MUCH

There are times that the stomach-to-brain feedback loop is not reliable. Studies show that the other mechanism that yoga exploits—the stomach stretch receptors turning off the brain's appetite producers—is highly sensitive to time of day. This diurnal variation fixes the feedback loop as maximally sensitive about noon and, as I've said, only one-quarter as effective at midnight. This means that insomniac eating is a very dangerous thing for those who are concerned about their waistlines. Many of the people who sleeplessly wander toward the fridge in the wee hours devour whole quarts of ice cream or all the leftovers.

But yoga can also be used to fall asleep before that midnight trip to the fridge. Because this feedback loop between the stretch receptors in your esophagus, stomach, and duodenum is so much less sensitive at midnight, nighttime eating should be kept to a minimum. When you can put yourself to sleep at night, the odds of this self-abuse go down.

As you will see, seven minutes of yoga that can be done in bed can also help you stay asleep, or fall back asleep after waking up in the middle of the night.

Here is an email I received about a week before turning this book in to the publisher:

Dear Loren,

I used your new leg stretch, breathed incorrectly a few times, and fell immediately into a four-hour deep sleep. I've thrown them [the sleeping medicine] away. . . .

Thanks for everything.
RS, Connecticut

The following yoga sequence can be completed entirely in bed. I have used this method many times with patients in my practice, and on the whole they are grateful. It may take a week or three for the beneficial sleep to occur on cue, but before very long, it almost always has the desired effect. After a while many people fall asleep before they finish it. I estimate the success rate at about 90 percent. There are three parts to it. One begins lying on one's back:

PART 1

Supta Padangusthasana I
(no good English translation)

Benefits and how it works: Certainly, this helps you sleep without disturbing anyone else. It also stretches your hamstrings without endangering an osteoporotic spine, and brings about a sense of calm bodily awareness that may reappear in the morning, on the other end of the pleasant journey of sleep. The stretch receptors in the hamstring muscles send relaxing signals to the parts of the brain and brain stem that promote relaxation.

Contraindications: Ischial bursitis, hamstring tear, adductor tear. People with sleep apnea should have someone watch them when they start, and periodically thereafter. GERD patients may want a bolster under their chests and heads; this entire procedure is not recommended during acute asthma or bronchitis episodes or severe upper respiratory tract infections.

Helpful hint: If it helps, keep a belt by your bedside. When using the belt, hold it in both hands, and walk up the belt with your hands to maintain straight elbows as much as possible. When you've gone as far as you can, and your elbows are straight, then pull down from your shoulders by bringing the shoulders back down to the bed in a rowing motion.

THE POSE

1. Lie supine (face up), legs straight out horizontally. Don't use a pillow.
2. Press the right leg down so the back of the knee is in contact with the bed, while raising the left thigh up to vertical, knee bent.
3. Then straighten the left knee, and either grasp the big toe of the left foot with the first two fingers of the left hand, grasp the foot with both hands, or hold each side of a belt that wraps around the elevated foot just behind the ball of the foot.
4. Grasp the right wrist with the opposite hand or walk your fingers up the belt as far as possible. In any event, extend your reach so that your elbows are straight and your shoulders come up *a little* off the bed.
5. Breathe in as you tighten both legs' quadriceps and draw your shoulders down to the bed, which will bring the left leg closer to your forehead.
6. Retighten your quadriceps to retain a straight leg.
7. Hold the pose for thirty seconds, then reverse the legs and repeat.

LESS CHALLENGING VARIATIONS:
VARIATION 1

1. If you cannot straighten the left knee, or if the left leg is not yet at ninety degrees, do the pose with the right leg bent, foot flat on the bed, until your hamstrings become more flexible. This will tilt your pelvis backward and stabilize it, giving more leeway to stretch the left leg and also stabilize your pelvis.

2. Even if your right leg remains bent, elongate it by stretching through your heel, sliding your foot out and away from yourself.

3. For either variation, press the upper sacrum down, which will properly tilt the pelvis to achieve the hamstring stretch.

4. The main action is to push your left thigh *away* from your upper body (which maintains the arch in the lower back), against the resistance of the belt pulling the foot *toward* you. Note: The goal is *not* to force the left leg or foot toward your head, which will cause you to round your lower back.

5. Once you have all the actions going—have achieved the pose as best you can—scan your body for unnecessary tension and release it, especially in the abdomen, shoulders, neck, and face. Then go through the same steps on the other side. This pose increases patience and steadfastness, and sets you up for the second part.

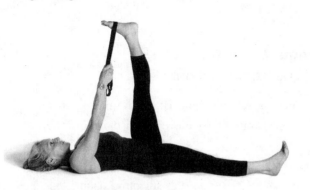

Supta Padangusthasana—
beginning

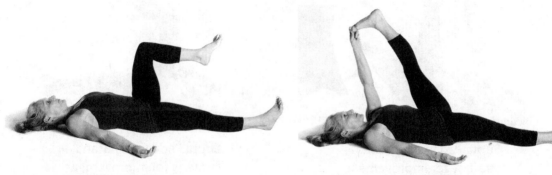

Supta Padangusthasana

Supta Padangusthasana—
adapted for tightness

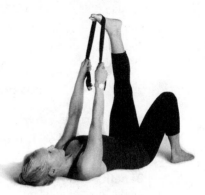

Supta Padangusthasana—with
tighter hamstrings

VARIATION 2

If you still cannot straighten your left leg when it is up beyond sixty degrees, then grasp the back of your left thigh with both hands as you elevate it, and make the knee as straight as possible.

Explanation: Sometimes the hamstrings are so tight that the leg goes up less than fifty degrees, even with the opposite leg's knee bent. In that case, the pulling is mostly straight against the bone, not the muscles. That situation demands holding the back of your thigh directly, and pulling the leg toward you from there. Keep the knee as straight as you can while doing so.

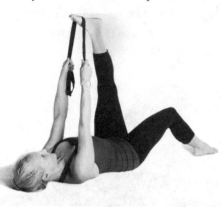

Supta Padangusthasana—
strategy for improvement

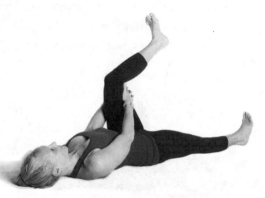

Supta Padangusthasana—
strategy for improvement

PART 2

Viloma I and II
(no good English translation)

These are breathing exercises known as Viloma I and II. As the names suggest, the exercise has two distinct sections. Don't move. Both can be done lying on your back.*

Benefits and how they work: I believe this breathing exercise separates the visceral and parietal pleura, two layers of tissue that surround each lung.

---

* To be fully informed, please see the video at www.YIP.guru.

These structures are richly invested with sensory fibers from the vagus nerve. Stimulating them calms down the "fight or flight" instinct, and promotes the "rest and digest" parasympathetic response so helpful for those seeking slumber.

Contraindications: People with sleep apnea should have someone watch them when they start and periodically thereafter. GERD patients may want a bolster under their upper back, neck, and head. This entire procedure is not recommended during acute asthma or bronchitis episodes or upper respiratory tract infections.

Helpful hint: When taking in the three parts of the breath in the first section, and exhaling in three parts in the second section, focus on keeping the velocity of the breath constant throughout each intake and expelling of air.

Viloma I

FOR THE FIRST SECTION:

1. Draw in a good breath. Keep your chest full—puffed out—by sustaining all the muscular effort that you used to inhale that air.
2. Then, without collapsing your chest at all, smoothly release all the air you comfortably can—again, keeping the chest large and puffy.
3. Rest for a moment with the air expelled, then slowly and smoothly take in approximately one-third of a complete breath. Stop again, still not using your throat or tongue as a stopper; instead, just still the diaphragm in its descent in your chest.
4. After a few moments, breathe in the second one-third of the air.
5. Again stop without closing off your throat.
6. After a few more seconds, take in the final one-third of air to fill your lungs up well.
7. Pause for a moment when your lungs are full, then exhale completely.
8. Now take a normal breath. The pressures in your chest affect the blood flow to the heart muscle itself, as well as the lungs and brain. You need a normal breath to reestablish these complex and critical rhythms.
9. Then repeat the above procedure, and after that take a normal breath.
10. Then repeat it yet a third time.

Take another normal breath, and proceed to do the complementary Viloma II:

Viloma II

FOR THE SECOND SECTION:

1. Puff out your chest with a good breath of air.
2. Gently and smoothly exhale one-third of the air you've just inhaled. Stop the exhalation just by halting the diaphragm's ascent, without using tongue or throat.
3. Pause for a few seconds and exhale the second one-third of the air.
4. Pause again, and after a few seconds, exhale completely.
5. Then take a normal breath.
6. Repeat the three-part exhalation procedure for two more breaths, being careful to take a normal breath between each of them.

You have completed the breathing part of the path to nighttime slumber. The third part is conceptual. It is one of the meditation techniques that derive from the Vairagya Tantric masters of Kashmir Shaivism.[3] They are meant to help center the individual and bring him or her closer to a universal consciousness.

There are nine concepts, to be contemplated for about half a minute each, in the same order every time you use them. Do not monitor the timing too closely, as that will distract you. The idea is to place the concept clearly before your mind and then watch it slowly fade from that heightened consciousness. Then you go on to the next concept. The first few times you use the concepts, you'll need to consult the place where they are written, but within a few days they'll be in your memory. The nine concepts are:

Love
Radiance
Unity
Health
Strength
Abundance

Wisdom
Light-as-air
Inner space

Reliably putting oneself to sleep is a step toward unifying the mind; it's what Patanjali, the author of the first yoga book, some two thousand years ago, alluded to when he wrote, "Yoga reduces mental inconstancy." It also raises self-confidence and actual enjoyment of life.*

---

* For more on sleeping, please see the video recording of my May 14, 2019, webinar at https://zoom.us/webinar/register/WN_1ar2AuCNRXmY-uvjWa5SnQ.

CHAPTER 10

From the Practical
to the Sublime

I'T'S NOT THAT WE don't have reasons to lose excessive or unwanted weight; there are plenty of reasons: health, looks, clothing fashions. But apparently those reasons are not strong enough, not persuasive for the vast numbers of overweight people in our country and across the world. Think not just about yourself but about all the people you know, and I am willing to wager there is more than one who professes the desire to become slimmer.

Why is eating so different from other natural functions? We don't need to coax people to breathe right—not too little, not too much. There is no great crusade encouraging us to drink enough water, or to go to the bathroom when we need to. What is so troublesome with eating? The bookstores aren't bulging with works on why you should scratch where and when it itches and then stop. Why is it so challenging when the desire is not to scratch an itch but to put just the right amount in one's stomach and leave it at that? As David Seymour, a political leader in New Zealand, has noted, "The strange reality of obesity is that it's an epidemic of choice. It's not brought by wayward mosquitos or by economic recession. It's brought to us by our own hand, in spite of decades of information campaigns on the value of exercise and healthy eating."

But that's a simplified story. Economic, social, educational, personal, and even political concerns make a great deal of difference in what we eat, when we eat, and, yes, how much we eat. Hormonal differences, energy-balance mechanisms, and other heritable traits are also involuntary weight-influencing factors. Possibly we are running into the uniting of evolutionary priorities and cultural imperatives. Those people who eat judiciously or are vegetarian do better than those who will eat anything that doesn't eat them first. But we are contending with a strong and instinctive tendency to consume, an inborn hunger as deep and indomitable as life itself.

Here in the United States, there has been a gigantic effort to motivate citizens to control their weight. Yet, in spite of the rational works on diet, the prodigious efforts of the pharmaceutical community, and the peer pressure generated by motivational meetings, e.g., Weight Watchers, as much as two-thirds of the nation remains overweight.

The looming specter of an early death doesn't even come close to being a big enough motivator. What you look like doesn't seem to do it for most people either. The price of food is often the trade-off of quality for quantity—junk food that adds to obesity with cheap, weight-enhancing ingredients like corn syrup, which can also fuel the growth of cancer.

It doesn't have to be that way. Like any other skill—like learning to add two and two, like becoming good at using a knife and fork or doing yoga—with practice, you can become better at being motivated. Understanding a little more about how to become more skilled will help.

First, not sleeping long enough or well enough and experiencing a lot of stress will interfere with your ability to stay on track with any plan, including an eating plan or a yoga program. You just may not have the energy or room in your mind to care as much as you need to if you're tired or nervous and cortisol and other fat-generating hormones are coursing through your veins. You need to care a lot if you're going to stick to a routine of fifteen-minutes-before-a-meal yoga and careful eating. So be good to yourself at bedtime, do yoga to help you go to sleep and stay asleep (see page 120–127), and remember that yoga reduces stress and increases calm.

If you have failed in the past, as so often happens, feeling guilty makes it more difficult to succeed the next time. As you've heard so many times in so many different contexts, take baby steps.

And when you *do* manage to succeed in leaving the table a little hungry or doing the yoga before a big meal every day for a week, give yourself credit. Acknowledge your success. It's important—even more important than avoiding feeling too bad when you slip up. Don't *just* pat yourself on the back; realistic assessment is best.

Science has shown that giving yourself a little reward just when you achieve your goal is like a beneficial shot in the arm. A reward can be anything, and it definitely doesn't have to be food. It can be listening to a song you like, looking at a tree, freshening up by sweeping a comb through your hair. The trick is to give yourself the reward immediately after you've earned it by forgoing that soft drink, for instance, and to reward yourself often. The better you do, the more rewards you will get and the better you will feel.[1]

HOW GOAL PROGRESS INFLUENCES REGULATORY FOCUS IN GOAL PURSUIT

Frequent rewards increase motivation. But you also need willpower. Experts agree that willpower—the strength to carry out your own wishes instead of giving in to your sometimes less-than-beneficial desires—weakens throughout the day. You will probably be more able to exercise your willpower earlier in the day. So, not only should you make every effort to sleep enough, after you rise in the morning be kind to yourself. You can give yourself a minute or two of rest here and there during every day so your willpower "muscle" doesn't get tired and peter out. Just close your eyes and breathe for a minute or two, and forget everything outside of your breath.

Rather than putting a lock on your refrigerator so you don't open it when you know you shouldn't, either during the day or late at night, cut yourself some slack. You may want to put something in your mouth, chew it up, and swallow it. You may know specifically what that thing is that you want that's on the second shelf in the fridge. You can acknowledge that craving to yourself; you can even smile at it. That doesn't mean you need to give in to it.

What you do regarding your eating is a choice you can and must make every time you feel you want to do something you know you will later regret. Instead of saying to yourself, "I can't have that ice cream in the freezer," you can say, "I am choosing not to have the ice cream because . . ." You have free will and you can use it. David Seymour's calling obesity an epidemic of choice has some truth in it. But that truth has an opposite side to its coin. Just as you can choose to be overweight, you can choose to slim down and to stay slim.

One trick that works for me and others is to put off gratification, just temporarily. If you're an ice-cream eater, you can say to yourself, "Yes, I'll have what's left in that pint of chocolate ice cream that's in the freezer because I just can't stand to be without it. But I won't have it right this minute. I'll wait five or ten minutes. Or I'll wait until tomorrow. Or I'll open the freezer right this very minute and throw it out." Of course, keeping temptation out of reach, even out of the house, is also a good strategy.

Which brings me to goal-setting. Obviously, when embarking on a weight-loss plan of any kind, you need to know where you're going. Be very specific when deciding what you want to accomplish. If you're vague, you're less likely to succeed. So write down your objectives. There are two parts to this goal-setting—short-term goals and long-term goals. Both are crucial to any weight-loss plan.

You don't need to know what you're doing today and every day for the next week, even every day for the next month. But avoiding gaining back weight you lost is part of a long-term goal. Actually, if you don't decide that the changes you're going to make—in how you eat, how you do yoga, how you sleep—are permanent, you will almost certainly fail. You really do need to commit to changing your life and your lifestyle, not just for now but for always.

What happens is that without a commitment to the future—probably to the future for as long as you live—you gradually become overconfident. You can keep up with radical changes for a while, for instance cutting out sweets completely. You may do very well that way, even lose weight you keep off for as long as a year or two. But then, insidiously, bit by bit, it's likely that you will revert to your old habits. That's really a place where yoga can come in and save the day.

As I've said so many times, a regular yoga practice is not only a physical thing. It's emotional and it's spiritual. After doing yoga regularly, even for a relatively short time, your appetite lessens; maybe even more important, your point of view changes. You see yourself differently. You see the world differently. You see food differently. You respect yourself and everything else more than you did before.

SPIRITUALITY

Spirituality is what you can get from yoga. In almost every known form, yoga works to unify the body, mind, and spirit. Practiced wisely and well and, above all, persistently, yoga silently guides you to walk through life as inside a gigantic cathedral: thrilled by each new sight and sound and smell, yet cognizant of the dimensions of your place in the whole pageant of space and time. It may sound overly grand, but even the casual practitioner finds her- or himself "one with the universe," balancing the seesaw of what is here-and-now and what has always been so. Yoga resolves the opposition of mind and body through simultaneously brightening our current perceptions and our awareness of what lies beyond all experience. That's the spiritual part. As Aristotle and Buddha might say in one voice: "It is a question of balance."

I am not focusing on meditation here but the practical matter of losing weight. What I am driving at? With yoga you can see and feel, palpably know, the sanctity of your body and its parts. As Carl Sagan both said and proved, we are made of stardust. In yoga you quickly see how this is compatible with Shakespeare's "We are the stuff that dreams are made on." Regular yoga practice can give you a reverence and respect for the world and for your own body as part of it, a sentiment strong enough to overcome the tendency to distort your body through overeating.

We have known this, in many different forms, for a long time—a very long time. It has been described in many ways and found along many different paths. It could be called "consciousness."

In the first chapter of *White Fang*, written almost a century ago, in 1924, author Jack London describes a harrowing dog-sled trip through the frozen Yukon in which a pack of starving wolves follows increasingly disabled dog-sledders through the forest. At last, only one man remains, with two dogs that cower beside him. They can go no farther. He builds a circular fire around himself and the dogs, and painstakingly moves the edges of the fire from tree to tree in order to secure fuel for it. He's tired and has been awake for days. The many wolves are audaciously close.

> As he piled wood on the fire he discovered an appreciation of his own
> body which he had never felt before. He watched his moving muscles

and was interested in the cunning mechanisms of his fingers by the light of the fire. He crooked his fingers slowly and repeatedly now one at a time, now all together, spreading them wide or making quick gripping movements. He studied the nail formation and prodded the fingertips now sharply and again softly, gauging the while the nerve sensations produced. It fascinated him, and he grew suddenly fond of the subtle flesh of his that worked so beautifully and smoothly and delicately. . . . Never had he been so fond of this body of his as now when his tenure of it was so precarious.[2]

This is how new yoga practitioners feel, especially those sensing the baleful gaze of medical probabilities that surround them and track them through their days as the watchful wolves do in this vignette. As with Jack London's musher, the more aware one is of the health hazards that surround obesity and overweight, the more astonishing becomes the phenomenon of life and the "cunning mechanisms" of the human body.

And this translates into what every one of us can experience today.

Eric Newman, MD, gained sixty pounds during his undergraduate years at the University of Maryland.

I had a scholarship to college and I ate a lot of cafeteria food. Very little salad but lots of mozzarella sticks and things like that. I kind of gained the Freshman Fifteen every year. I didn't know anything about healthy eating. I mean I did know there were certain foods that were good for you but I didn't actually realize that eating those foods could make you feel better and that, for instance, eating other less healthy things could make you feel tired.

I tried yoga and did it for about a year in college. I think that hot yoga and yoga in general have something really important. . . . I do believe that yoga teaches you to be more mindful. So you'll eat better. And you'll notice that if you eat healthier, you'll feel better. I wanted to lose weight and it happened gradually.

I was definitely overweight, borderline obese. I noticed I had more energy when I was doing yoga and I wanted to lose a little bit of weight. I didn't have it in mind to get down to 155—I thought I might lose twenty pounds or so. It's been gradual over ten years to where I am now, and where I am now, I might even be able to gain a little weight. I've lost sixty pounds.

Every day, beginning when I wake up, I do some yoga. Often I do it in bed . . . and I meditate. . . . I do Yoga Nidra [a powerful relaxation technique related to the "relaxation response"] in bed before I get up. Sometimes I meditate on the bus on the way to work. All day, every once in a while, I close my eyes and try to be mindful. And three to five days a week I take a class. My favorite poses are backbends, but I like them all.

Matters of the spirit are formidable motivators. We can see this in our own times in those who give their lives (or even take the lives of others) for what they conceive as a spiritual (or religious) cause. Well, if a spiritual impulse can be strong enough to compel someone to do something as unspiritual as kill, then it might be up to the task of countering the propensity to eat and keep right on eating.

The great religions of this world, and many of the lesser-known ones, are replete with beautiful and profound stories. Yet the elaborate and so very well-known traditions and rituals that accompany the hierarchical structure of so many religious orders do not attract our universal admiration. They are often seen as fusions of business, politics, brainwashing, and fiction. But still, the spiritual impulse is within us, a yearning for something to revere, something we may reasonably seek.

Yoga may not be the only thing that does this, that prompts you to receive your experience as an infinitesimal slice of a vast and limitless whole, but yoga does help you, almost compels you, to live in the skein of "nows" that are part and parcel of eternity. To see with your mind what you feel in your body . . . a sweet reasonableness that sweeps you beyond the mind and body into a spiritual place. This is what my teacher, B.K.S. Iyengar, meant when he said, "My body is my temple." It is actually the place of spiritual worship that goes well beyond flesh and blood, because when you sense the mind and body united, it takes you places that neither can by itself.

A few years ago I gave a talk in Haridwar, a sacred city in northern India. It was a milestone anniversary, so my wife and I made a vacation out of it.

As our time was limited it seemed best to avoid the long trip to Pune, where Mr. Iyengar was then still practicing. At times I felt such remorse: "How can I come all this way and not see my teacher?" But then, walking down from the stage directly after my talk, a miracle occurred: Coming up the stairs was Mr. Iyengar! We recognized each other at once, and after the briefest of greetings I asked, "If you had one more thing to tell me, what would it be?" He paused for what seemed like an eon. He drew a breath and replied, "You only rent your body."

That was the last time we met. I take what he said to emphasize that we, both our bodies and everything that they are heir to, are part of the greater universe. Even our bodies we do not own. We should care for them with the selfless altruism of a respectful tenant.

It seems clear that all the books and all the reasons, medical, social, cultural—all good reasons—simply do not add up to enough motivation to deter the forces that cause overweight in the long term. Today the grisly truth is that, though there are ways to avoid it, and I have enumerated some of them in these pages, many dieters regain the weight they have lost within a few years.

Here lies the mismatch: Intellectual and practical persuasion are not equal to the task of producing a motivation strong enough and long enough to accomplish an obviously desirable goal: normal weight. The fiery harangue, delivered in advertisements, through TED talks, or from the myriad portals of the medical community, have had a feeble and time-limited effect. After a while, as one patient put it, "their words are dead birds," falling to the ground before reaching a place where they might roost and propagate. The diets become tiresome, and either the people on the diet, their closest associates, or their circumstances cannot support the effort for very long. Either the motivation is not strong enough or the task is too arduous. Ennui sets in, and is closely followed by indifference. Then the ancient impulse to self-nourish takes over again.

Yoga was recently added to the UNESCO list of Intangible Cultural Heritage. Yoga—without a central committee, without a governing body or a clergy of any kind, with never a conquering army enforcing its precepts on anyone, monotheistic but nonsectarian—is valued by many tens of millions of people, who come to it in innumerable ways. Once they do, most will stay for the same reason: They value it for what it does within them. UNESCO tweeted, "Designed to help individuals build self-realization, ease any suffering they may be experiencing and allow for a state of liberation, [yoga] is practiced by the young and old without discriminating against gender, class or religion."[3]

In my assessment, when people talk of things spiritual, they mean faith. But if you analyze what *faith* means, you may be surprised. Faith is belief; it is trust.[4] It is the conviction that "God is on your side," be it in a fox-hole, while giving birth, or when pursuing a dream or a career. In Western and Middle Eastern monotheistic terms, faith is belief in an all-powerful "Backer." As such, it is also an inner persuasion that one will succeed. And that is really the equivalent of having faith in oneself. You could even say strong self-confidence. Faith in these terms is still spiritual; it is the belief in what one can do in the future. Seen this way, faith is belief in what at this moment cannot be known with certainty, since the proof of it lies beyond any evidence that the present can possibly offer. The present gives, by definition, insufficient data by which a finite individual can predict the future.

This is the untenable position in which we find ourselves—we and any creature rational enough to anticipate tomorrow. "Life is what happens while you're making plans." Faith in these terms is *trust*, possibly trust in a supreme being, someone who can make things come out right, in this case functioning as a liaison between one's aspirations and one's confidence that those aspirations can be achieved. But no matter, it comes to the same thing: It is conviction that a person can do what he or she proposes to do. Here are Jesse Ruggiere's thoughts.

> While everyone is different, I am living proof that yoga is *extremely* effective when it comes to lasting weight loss. When I first rolled out the mat seven years ago, I was eighty-five pounds overweight. I was unhealthy, unhappy, and fueled by a passion for binge-drinking and pizza. When I first announced my mission to lose weight through yoga, I remember people laughing at me. "Yoga doesn't help with weight loss! You have to bust your butt in the gym to get *real* results," people told me.
>
> Less than one year later, after practicing yoga six to seven days per week, I lost a total of eighty-five pounds.

When you embark upon a yoga journey, you will begin to see things in a new light. Yoga transforms you from the inside out—and typically in that order. When the soul is awakened through yoga practice, the things that used to please you just no longer cut it. When you are in touch with your spiritual nature, you begin to realize that life has deeper meaning. You come to understand that destructive habits no longer serve your ultimate goal. This awakening directly affects weight loss because it encourages the elimination of unhealthy actions.

Jennifer B. Niles, author and founder of The Organic Transformation, says it several times: Respecting yourself, trusting yourself, having confidence, is exactly what yoga brings to so many people. Yoga accomplishes this in subtle ways: Through the disciplines of *asana* (doing the poses), *Pranayama* (breathing exercises), and meditation, yoga manages to unify body, mind, and spirit. It does not matter whether you take *spirit* to mean "high-spirited" or, more religiously, "Spirit." Whatever you identify as spiritual goes beyond what we know, transcends in the sense of being yet unproven, and is, as they say, "a matter of faith." But this ethereal thing is nonetheless one of the most powerful forces known to humankind.

Possibly by unifying the diverse currents of biology, intellect, and intention, yoga succeeds in making you aware, first, that your spirit is alive; second, that you, the person, have greater intrinsic value than you ever suspected; and finally, that your value translates into caring for yourself just as well as caring for other people. That means caring for yourself both in the sense that friends care for each other, and in the sense in which people care for a rented property.

What I am promising you is that if you take yoga to heart, at first tentatively, rationally, and later with serious striving, you will experience substantially greater self-regard, self-respect, and, finally, almost transcendentally greater commitment to continuing to make yourself better. So yes, yoga in itself has special means to help you lose weight—an uncompromisingly strong and personally ethical means.

A regular yoga practice is a worthwhile means to a somewhat pedestrian goal: lasting weight loss. Yoga can do this in a number of ways. First, physiologically: engaging your body in such a way as to inhibit your appetite and improve your metabolism "off the mat." Second, by making visible the sacred nature of your life, and of life itself, enabling your will to lead you into a more beautiful and balanced life. Third, by gifting you a clarity of mind and steadfastness of spirit that enable you to perceive your wants versus your needs—what is good versus what is pleasant—and, without further judgment, to act in your own behalf.

I dearly hope that this book will furnish you with enough motivation and enough means to accomplish the goal of losing weight. Unlike medication, surgery, and diets, yoga can be embraced throughout every life it tends to lengthen, broaden, and make more profound.

Acknowledgments

THANK YOU TO my patient editor, Jill Bialosky; to supportive Ellen Levine; and to Sarah Johnson for her help with the manuscript. For the close reading and advice given us on the manuscript, we thank Jessica Friedman. We are grateful to Drew Weitman for her kind responsiveness. We, and you, the reader, must thank Molly Heron for her intuitive and graceful design of the book. Beautiful pose demonstrations in these pages were done by Carrie Owerko, Lara Benusis, and Liz Larson, who spent hours getting everything just right. Most of all, gratitude to B.K.S. Iyengar, not only for his teachings, but for his inspiration, which continues always.

Alphabetical List of Poses

Poses by Chapter

Glossary

Ankylosing spondylitis: A genetically determined form of arthritis in which the vertebral bodies become fused, usually before thirty years of age, after which time movement within the spine is impossible.

Anterior cruciate ligament (ACL): The ACL connects the back of the femur to the front of the tibial plateau at the knee, restricting forward movement of the shin with respect to the femur.

Anterolisthesis: The sliding forward of one vertebra with respect to the one below it.

Aortic aneurism: Swelling of the aorta, usually indicating a rupture in the stronger muscular walls of that vessel. Generally in the abdomen, but may be more rostral.

Arthritis: Inflammation of a joint, generally either rheumatoid, an autoimmune condition, or osteoarthritic, also inflammatory, but more related to trauma or microtrauma. Other types include gouty, bacterial, and pigmented villonodular.

Bariatric surgery: Surgical reduction of the capacity of the stomach, through frank resection, belting, or other similar procedures.

Bursa: Pouch or potential space usually between two muscles or between a muscle or tendon and a bone.

Bursitis: Inflammation and swelling of a bursa.

Cauda equina: The strands of nerve rootlets that carry signals below the conus medullaris, generally at T12–L1, but sometimes one level higher or lower.

Central spinal canal: Long tubular structure through which nervous tissue passes, connecting the brain to the body and vice versa.

Chondromalacia patellae: Significant reduction of the cartilage of the kneecap that interfaces with the femoral condyles and the tibial plateau.

Coccygodynia: Pain stemming from the coccyx. Frequently the coccyx is displaced to one side or forward or backward.

Colostomy: Opening from the colon through the skin, frequently emptying its contents into a colostomy bag.

Colostomy bag: Often used temporarily following colon or rectal surgery.

Compression fracture: Spinal vertebral fracture in which the front of the superior plate of the vertebra is depressed, so the vertebra resembles a wedge. Frequently seen in osteoporosis.

Cotrel-Dubousset: Surgical wiring procedure for scoliosis, giving a three-dimensional contour to the repaired spine, but restricting its movement considerably.

Degenerative joint disease (DJD): Arthritis. Generally osteoarthritis is meant, not rheumatoid.

Diaphragm: Large muscular structure attached to the spine and ribs that contracts downward to cause inhalation, and relaxes upward for exhalation.

Dislocation: When the component bones of a joint are not in the proper alignment.

Distal: Adjective meaning far from the center of the body, as opposed to *proximal*, meaning close to it.

Duodenum: The first part of the small intestine, into which the stomach empties.

Esophagus: The part of the digestive tract below (distal to) the pharynx and above (proximal to) the stomach.

Facet arthritis: Degenerative joint disease affecting the vertebral facets, often causing swelling into the central canal.

Femur: Bone between the hip and the knee.

Gastroesophageal junction: Sphincter between the esophagus and the stomach.

Greater trochanter: Lateral projection of the proximal femur just as the bone angles inward toward the pelvis. Many muscles attach to it.

Harrington rod: Surgical treatment for scoliosis in which the vertebrae are fused and attached to a rod to reduce the curve(s).

Herniated nucleus pulposus (HNP) (herniated disc): Break in the outer ring of an intervertebral disc (annulus fibrosus) through which inner gelatinous material may ooze (nucleus pulposus).

Hyperlordosis: Excessive concave backward arching of the lumbar spine.

Ischial bursitis: Inflammation of the bursa at the ischial bone.

Kyphosis: Forward arching of any part of the spine, convex when seen from the back.

Lateral: To the side.

Lateral listhesis: Slippage of a vertebral body to the right or left relative to the vertebra beneath it.

Lateral meniscal tear (LMT): Pathological break in the cartilage of the lateral part of the knee joint.

Lordosis: Arching of any part of the spine that is concave when seen from the back.

Medial meniscal tear (MMT): Pathological break in the cartilage of the medial part of the knee joint.

Osteoporosis: Bone mineral density 2.5 standard deviations below the norm seen in twenty-five- to thirty-year-old women in the hip, femur, or any lumbar vertebra.

Ostomies: Openings through the skin allowing intestinal contents to be emptied, e.g., colostomy (from the colon), iliostomy (from the ileum).

Pelvic diaphragm: Muscles of the lower pelvis that hold its contents upward, e.g., levator ani.

Plantar fasciitis: Inflammation or tearing of the tough fascia that connects the bases of the toes with the heel.

Posterior cruciate ligament (PCL): The PCL connects the front of the femur to the back of the tibial plateau at the knee, restricting backward movement of the shin with respect to the femur.

Pregnancy trimester: Trimesters divide the nine-month period of normal pregnancy into three-month segments.

Quadratus lumborum (QL): Large rectangular muscles connecting the posterior lower ribs with the posterior pelvic rim.

Retro: Latin prefix meaning "after" or "behind."

Retrolisthesis: Backward sliding of a vertebral body with respect to the one below it.

Rotator cuff syndrome (RCS): Partial or full tear of the supraspinatus, infraspinatus, teres minor, or subscapularis muscles, most commonly the supraspinatus.

Sacroiliac joint derangement: Improper alignment of the sacrum with the iliac bones on either side of it.

Scoliosis: Sideward curvature of the spine of more than ten degrees.

Spinal fixator: Anything surgically placed in or adjacent to the spine that substantially limits the motion of the vertebrae.

Spinal stenosis: Narrowing of the central spinal canal.

Subluxation: Minor misalignment of a joint.

Torque: Twisting force.

Total knee replacement (TKR): Surgical substitution of artificial components that supplant the weight-bearing structures of the knee joint.

Vertebral compression fracture: Spinal vertebral fracture in which the front of the superior plate of the vertebra is depressed, so the vertebra resembles a wedge. Frequently seen in osteoporosis.

Vertebral displacement: Misalignment of one or more spinal vertebrae.

Wedge fracture: Spinal vertebral fracture in which the front of the superior plate of the vertebra is depressed, so the vertebra resembles a wedge. Frequently seen in osteoporosis.

Notes

Introduction: **The Yogic Approach**

1. For example, E. Amy Janke, Elizabeth Jones, Christina M. Hopkins, Madelyn Ruggieri, and Alesha Hruska, "Catastrophizing and Anxiety Sensitivity Mediate the Relationship between Persistent Pain and Emotional Eating," *Appetite* 103 (August 2016): 64–71; Suzan A. Haidar, N. K. de Vries, Mirey Karavetian, and Rola El-Rassi, "Stress, Anxiety, and Weight Gain among University and College Students: A Systematic Review," *Journal of the Academy of Nutrition and Dietetics* 118, no. 2 (2018): 261–74; Jeni Matthews, Jennifer Huberty, Jenn Leiferman, and Matthew Buman, "Psychosocial Predictors of Gestational Weight Gain and the Role of Mindfulness," *Midwifery* 56 (January 2018): 86–93.

Chapter 1 **Tangible and Intangible Yoga Influences**

1. KayLoni L. Olson and Charles F. Emery, "Mindfulness and Weight Loss: A Systematic Review," *Psychosomatic Medicine* 77, no. 1 (2015): 59–67.

Chapter 2 **Benefits for Conditions Related to Overweight**

1. Herbert Benson, John F. Beary, and Mark P. Carol, "The Relaxation Response," *Psychiatry* 37, no. 1 (1974): 37–46; Rashmi Yadav, Raj Kumar Yadav, Rajesh Khadgawat, and Nalin Mehta, "Beneficial Effects of a 12-Week Yoga-Based Lifestyle Intervention on Cardio-Metabolic Risk Factors in Subjects with Pre-hypertension or Hypertension," *Journal of Hypertension* 34, e-Supplement 1 (2016): e252.

2. Kim E. Innes and Heather K. Vincent, "The Influence of Yoga-Based Programs on Risk Profiles in Adults with Type 2 Diabetes Mellitus: A Systematic Review," *Evidence-Based Complementary and Alternative Medicine* 4, no. 4 (2007): 469–86; Maria G. Araneta, Matthew A. Allison, Elizabeth Barrett-Connor, and Alka M. Kanaya, "Evidence Based Diabetes Management" (paper presented at the 73rd Session of American Diabetes Association, Chicago, IL, June 21–25, 2013).

3. Kumar Sarvottam, Dipti Magan, Raj Kumar, Nalin Mehta, and Sushil C. Mahapatra, "Adiponectin, Interleukin-6, and Cardiovascular Disease Risk Factors Are Modified by a Short-Term Yoga-Based Lifestyle Intervention in Overweight and Obese Men," *Journal of Alternative and Complementary Medicine* 19, no. 5 (2013): 397–402; Ramesh Lal Bijlani, R. P. Vempati, Raj Kumar Yadav, Rooma Basu Ray, Vani Gupta, Ratna Sharma, Nalin J. Mehta, and Sushil Chandra Mahapatra, "A Brief but Comprehensive Lifestyle Education Program Based on Yoga Reduces Risk Factors for Cardiovascular Disease and Diabetes Mellitus," *Journal of Alternative and Complementary Medicine* 11, no. 2 (2005): 267–74; Donald A. Williamson, "Fifty Years of Behavioral/Lifestyle Interventions for Overweight and Obesity: Where Have We Been and Where Are We Going?," *Obesity* 25, no. 11 (2017): 1867–75.

4. Zu-Yao Yang, Hui-Bin Zhong, Chen Mao, Jin-Qiu Yuan, Ya-Fang Huang, Xin-Yin Wu, Yuan-Mei Gao, and Jin-Ling Tang, "Yoga for Asthma," *Cochrane Database of Systematic Reviews* 4 (April 27, 2016). For example, see Sharon Lack, Roy Brown, and Patricia A. Kinser, "An Integrative Review of Yoga and Mindfulness-Based Approaches for Children and Adolescents with Asthma," *Journal of Pediatric Nursing* 52 (May–June 2020): 76–81; Holger Cramer, Paul Posadzki, Gustav Dobos, and Jost Langhorst, "Yoga for Asthma: A Systematic Review and Meta-analysis," *Annals of Allergy, Asthma & Immunology* 112, no. 6 (2014): 503–10.

5. See, e.g., Vicki A. Freedenberg, Pamela S. Hinds, and Erika Friedmann, "Mindfulness-Based Stress Reduction and Group Support Decrease Stress in Adolescents with Cardiac Diagnoses: A Randomized Two-Group Study," *Pediatric Cardiology* 38, no. 7 (2017): 1415–25; Debbie Cohen and Raymond R. Townsend, "Yoga and Hypertension," *Journal of Clinical Hypertension* 9, no. 19 (October 2007): 800–801; Holger Cramer, Heidemarie Haller, Romy Lauche, Nico Steckhan, Andreas Michalsen, and Gustav Dobos, "A Systematic Review and Meta-analysis of Yoga for Hypertension," *American Journal of Hypertension* 27, no. 9 (September 2014): 1146–51.

6. L. Susan Wieland and Nancy Santesso, "A Summary of a Cochrane Review: Yoga Treatment for Chronic Non-specific Low Back Pain," *European Journal of Integrative Medicine* 11 (2017): 39–40; L. Susan Wieland, Nicole Skoetz, Karen Pilkington, Ramaprabhu Vempati, Christopher R. D'Adamo, and Brian M. Berman, "Yoga Treatment for Chronic Non-specific Low Back Pain," *Cochrane Database of Systematic Reviews* 2017, no. 1 (January 12, 2017).

7. Alejandro Chaoul, Kathrin Milbury, Amy Spelman, Karen Basen-Engquist, Martica H. Hall, Qi Wei, Ya-Chen Tina Shih, Banu Arun, Vicente Valero, George H. Perkins, Gildy V. Babiera, Tenzin Wangyal, Rosalinda Engle, Carol A. Harrison, Yisheng Li, and Lorenzo Cohen, "Randomized Trial of Tibetan Yoga in Patients with Breast Cancer Undergoing Chemotherapy," *Cancer* 124, no. 1 (2017): 36–45.

8. Yi-Hsueh Lu, Bernard Rosner, Gregory Chang, and Loren M. Fishman, "Twelve-Minute Daily Yoga Regimen Reverses Osteoporotic Bone Loss," *Topics in Geriatric Rehabilitation* 32, no. 2 (2016): 81–87.

9. Lesley Ward, Simon Stebbings, Josie Athens, Daniel Cherkin, and G. David Baxter, "Yoga for the Management of Pain and Sleep in Rheumatoid Arthritis: A Pilot Randomized Controlled Trial," *Musculoskeletal Care* 16, no. 1 (2017): 39–47.

10. Ledetra Bridges and Manoj Sharma, "The Efficacy of Yoga as a Form of Treatment for Depression," *Journal of Evidence-Based Complementary & Alternative Medicine* 22, no. 4 (2017): 1010–28.

11. Loren M. Fishman, Erik J. Groessl, and Karen J. Sherman, "Serial Case Reporting Yoga for Idiopathic and Degenerative Scoliosis," *Global Advances in Health and Medicine* 3, no. 5 (2014): 16–21.

12. Bridges and Sharma, "Efficacy of Yoga."

13. Loren M. Fishman, Allen Wilkins, Caroline Konnoth, Sarah Schmidhofer, Tova Ovadia, and Bernard Rosner, "Yoga-Based Maneuver Effectively Treats Rotator Cuff Syndrome," *Topics in Geriatric Rehabilitation* 27, no. 2 (2011): 151–61. See https://sciatica.org under "Events Upcoming and Ongoing" for more details.

14. Frida Hylander, Maria Johansson, Daiva Daukantaitė, and Kai Ruggeri, "Yin Yoga and Mindfulness: A Five Week Randomized Controlled Study Evaluating the Effects of the YOMI Program on Stress and Worry," *Anxiety, Stress & Coping* 30, no. 4 (2017): 365–78; Edgar Toschi-Dias, Eleonora Tobaldini, Monica Solbiati, Giorgio Costantino, Roberto Sanlorenzo, Stefania Doria, Floriana Irtelli, Claudio Mencacci, and Nicola Montano, "Sudarshan

Kriya Yoga Improves Cardiac Autonomic Control in Patients with Anxiety-Depression Disorders," *Journal of Affective Disorders* 214 (2017): 74–80.

15. Robert E. Cushing and Kathryn L. Braun, "Mind-Body Therapy for Military Veterans with Post-Traumatic Stress Disorder: A Systematic Review," *Journal of Alternative and Complementary Medicine* 24, no. 2 (2017): 106–14.

16. Devon Brunner, Amitai Abramovitch, and Joseph Etherton, "A Yoga Program for Cognitive Enhancement," *PLOS One* 12, no. 8 (2017): e0182366.

17. Mrithunjay Rathore, Soumitra Trivedi, Jessy Abraham, and Manisha B. Sinha, "Anatomical Correlation of Core Muscle Activation in Different Yogic Postures," *International Journal of Yoga* 10, no. 2 (2017): 59–66.

18. Paul D. Smith, Paul Mross, and Nate Christopher, "Development of a Falls Reduction Yoga Program for Older Adults: A Pilot Study," *Complementary Therapies in Medicine* 31 (2017): 118–26; Savitha Subramaniam and Tanvi Bhatt, "Effect of Yoga Practice on Reducing Cognitive-Motor Interference for Improving Dynamic Balance Control in Healthy Adults," *Complementary Therapies in Medicine* 30 (2017): 30–35.

19. Melissa Mazor, Jeannette Q. Lee, Anne Peled, Sarah Zerzan, Chetan Irwin, Margaret A. Chesney, Katherine Serrurier, Hani Sbitany, Anand Dhruva, Devorah Sacks, and Betty Smoot, "The Effect of Yoga on Arm Volume, Strength, and Range of Motion in Women at Risk for Breast Cancer–Related Lymphedema," *Journal of Alternative and Complementary Medicine* 24, no. 2 (2017): 154–60.

20. Susannah H. Hartnoll and T. David Punt, "Yoga Practice Is Associated with Superior Motor Imagery Performance," *International Journal of Yoga Therapy* 27, no. 1 (2017): 81–86; B. R. Raghavendra and Shirley Telles, "Performance in Attentional Tasks Following Meditative Focusing and Focusing without Meditation," *Ancient Science of Life* 32, no. 1 (2012): 49–53.

21. Fereshteh Jahdi, Fatemeh Sheikhan, Hamid Haghani, Bahare Sharifi, Azizeh Ghaseminejad, Mahshad Khodarahmian, and Nicole Rouhana, "Yoga during Pregnancy: The Effects on Labor Pain and Delivery Outcomes (a Randomized Controlled Trial)," *Complementary Therapies in Clinical Practice* 27 (2017): 1–4.

22. Jin Lee, Ha-na Yoo, and Byoung-Hee Lee, "Effects of Augmented Reality–Based Otago Exercise on Balance, Gait, and Physical Factors in Elderly Women to Prevent Falls: A Randomized Controlled Trial," *Journal of Physical Therapy Science* 19, no. 9 (2017): 1586–89.

23. Rui F. Afonso, Joana B. Balardin, Sara Lazar, João R. Sato, Nadja Igarashi,

Danilo F. Santaella, Shirley S. Lacerda, Edson Amaro Jr., and Elisa H. Kozasa, "Greater Cortical Thickness in Elderly Female Yoga Practitioners: A Cross-Sectional Study," *Frontiers in Aging Neuroscience* 9 (June 20, 2017): 201.

24. Shirley Telles, Elisa Kozasa, Luciano Bernardi, and Marc Cohen, "Yoga and Rehabilitation: Physical, Psychological, and Social," *Evidence-Based Complementary and Alternative Medicine* 2013 (2013): 624758.

25. Shirley Telles, Bangalore N. Gangadhar, and Kavita D. Chandwani, "Lifestyle Modification in the Prevention and Management of Obesity," *Journal of Obesity* 2016 (2016): 581–601.

Chapter 3 Do You Really Need to Lose Weight?

1. Sabrina Youkhana, Catherine M. Dean, Moa Wolff, Catherine Sherrington, and Anne Tiedemann, "Yoga-Based Exercise Improves Balance and Mobility in People Aged 60 and Over: A Systematic Review and Meta-analysis," *Age and Ageing* 45, no. 1 (January 2016): 21–29.

Chapter 4 Real People Get Thinner

1. Géraldine M. Camilleri, Caroline Méjean, France Bellisle, Serge Hercberg, and Sandrine Péneau, "Mind-Body Practice and Body Weight Status in a Large Population-Based Sample of Adults," *American Journal of Preventive Medicine* 50, no. 4 (2016): e101–9; Shirley Telles, Sachin Kr. Sharma, Arti Yadav, Nilkamal Singh, and Acharya Balkrishna, "A Comparative Controlled Trial Comparing the Effects of Yoga and Walking for Overweight and Obese Adults," *Medical Science Monitor* 20 (2014): 894–904; *Yoga Journal* and Yoga Alliance in cooperation with Ipsos Public Affairs, *2016 Yoga in America Study*, https://www.yogaalliance.org/Portals/0/2016%20Yoga%20in%20America%20Study%20RESULTS.pdf; KayLoni L. Olson and Charles F. Emery, "Mindfulness and Weight Loss: A Systematic Review," *Psychosomatic Medicine* 77, no. 1 (2015): 59–67.

2. Shawn N. Katterman, Brighid M. Kleinman, Megan M. Hood, Lisa M. Nackers, and Joyce A. Corsica, "Mindfulness Meditation as an Intervention for Binge Eating, Emotional Eating, and Weight Loss: A Systematic Review," *Eating Behaviors* 15, no. 2 (2014): 197–204.

3. National Institute of Diabetes and Digestive and Kidney Diseases (NIDDK), "Overweight & Obesity Statistics," National Institutes of Health, August

2017, http://www.niddk.nih.gov/health-information/health-statistics/Pages/overweight-obesity-statistics.aspx#a.

4. NIDDK, "Overweight & Obesity Statistics."

5. *Yoga Journal* and Yoga Alliance, *2016 Yoga in America Study*.

Chapter 5 How Yoga Works Deep Inside Your Body

1. *Yoga Journal* and Yoga Alliance in cooperation with Ipsos Public Affairs, *2016 Yoga in America Study*, https://www.yogaalliance.org/Portals/0/2016%20Yoga%20in%20America%20Study%20RESULTS.pdf.

2. *Yoga Journal* and Yoga Alliance, *2016 Yoga in America Study*.

3. Romy Lauche, Jost Langhorst, Myeong Soo Lee, Gustav Dobos, and Holger Cramer, "A Systematic Review and Meta-analysis on the Effects of Yoga on Weight-Related Outcomes," *Preventive Medicine* 87 (2016): 213–32.

4. Janice K. Kiecolt-Glaser, Lisa M. Christian, Rebecca Andridge, Beom Seuk Hwang, William B. Malarkey, Martha A. Belury, Charles F. Emery, and Ronald Glaser, "Adiponectin, Leptin, and Yoga Practice," *Physiology & Behavior* 107, no. 5 (2012): 809–13; Amanda J. Page, James A. Slattery, Catherine Milte, Rhianna Laker, Tracey O'Donnell, Camilla Dorian, Stuart M. Brierly, and L. Ashley Blackshaw, "Ghrelin Selectively Reduces Mechanosensitivity of Upper Gastrointestinal Vagal Afferents," *American Journal of Physiology: Gastrointestinal and Liver Physiology* 292, no. 5 (2007): G1376–84.

5. Stefania Carmagnola, Paolo Cantù, and Roberto Penagini, "Mechanoreceptors of the Proximal Stomach and Perception of Gastric Distension," *American Journal of Gastroenterology* 100, no. 8 (2005): 1704–10.

6. M. M. Kutateladze and Aleksandre Asatiani, "Role of Gastric Mechanoreceptivity in Formation of Food Satiety" (article in Russian), *Georgian Medical News* 121 (2005): 78–81.

7. Stephen J. Kentish, Claudine L. Frisby, David J. Kennaway, Gary A. Wittert, and Amanda J. Page, "Circadian Variation in Gastric Vagal Afferent Mechanosensitivity," *Journal of Neuroscience* 33, no. 49 (2013): 19238–42; Carlos Celis-Morales, Donald M. Lyall, Yibing Guo, Lewis Steell, Daniel Llanas, Joey Ward, Daniel F. Mackay, Stephany M. Biello, Mark E. S. Bailey, Jill P. Pell, and Jason M. R. Gill, "Sleep Characteristics Modify the Association of Genetic Predisposition with Obesity and Anthropometric Measurements in

119,679 UK Biobank Participants," *American Journal of Clinical Nutrition* 105, no. 4 (2017): 980–90.

8. Kumar Sarvottam, Dipti Magan, Raj Kumar, Nalin Mehta, and Sushil C. Mahapatra, "Adiponectin, Interleukin-6, and Cardiovascular Disease Risk Factors Are Modified by a Short-Term Yoga-Based Lifestyle Intervention in Overweight and Obese Men," *Journal of Alternative and Complementary Medicine* 19, no. 5 (2013): 397–402; Celis-Morales et al., "Sleep Characteristics Modify the Association of Genetic Predisposition"; Lisa M. Jaremka, Martha A. Belury, Rebecca R. Andridge, William B. Malarkey, Ronald Glaser, Lisa Christian, Charles F. Emery, and Janice K. Kiecolt-Glaser, "Interpersonal Stressors Predict Ghrelin and Leptin Levels in Women," *Psychoneuroendocrinology* 48 (2014): 178–88.

9. Christoph Handschin and Bruce M. Spiegelman, "The Role of Exercise and PGC1α in Inflammation and Chronic Disease," *Nature* 454, no. 7203 (2008): 463–69.

10. This ability of PGC-1alpha has been challenged in the literature. Glenn C. Rowe, Riyad El-Khoury, Ian S. Patten, Pierre Rustin, and Zolt Arany, "PGC-1α Is Dispensable for Exercise-Induced Mitochondrial Biogenesis in Skeletal Muscle," *PLOS One* 7, no. 7 (2012): e41817.

11. Elizabeth H. Blackburn, Elissa S. Epel, and Jue Lin, "Human Telomere Biology: A Contributory and Interactive Factor in Aging, Disease Risks, and Protection," *Science* 350, no. 6265 (2015): 1193–98.

12. Jon Kabat-Zinn, *Full Catastrophe Living: Using the Wisdom of Your Body and Mind to Face Stress, Pain and Illness,* rev. ed. (New York: Bantam Books, 2013); Rainbow T. H. Ho, Jessie S. M. Chan, Chong-Wen Wang, Benson W. M. Lau, Kwok Fai So, Li Ping Yuen, Jonathan S. T. Sham, and Cecilia L. W. Chan, "A Randomized Controlled Trial of Qigong Exercise on Fatigue Symptoms, Functioning, and Telomerase Activity in Persons with Chronic Fatigue or Chronic Fatigue Syndrome," *Annals of Behavioral Medicine* 44, no. 2 (2012): 160–70; Elissa S. Epel, E. Puterman, J. Lin, E. H. Blackburn, P. Y. Lum, N. D. Beckmann, J. Zhu, E. Lee, A. Gilbert, R. A. Rissman, R. E. Tanzi, and E. E. Schadt, "Meditation and Vacation Effects Have an Impact on Disease-Associated Molecular Phenotypes," *Translational Psychiatry* 6, no. 8 (2016): e880.

13. Dean Ornish, Jue Lin, June M. Chan, Elissa Epel, Colleen Kemp, Gerdi Weidner, Ruth Marlin, Steven J. Frenda, Mark Jesus M. Magbanua, Jennifer Daubenmier, Ivette Estay, Nancy K. Hills, Nita Chainani-Wu, Peter

R. Carroll, and Elizabeth H. Blackburn, "Effect of Comprehensive Lifestyle Changes on Telomerase Activity and Telomere Length in Men with Biopsy-Proven Low-Risk Prostate Cancer: Five-Year Follow-Up of a Descriptive Pilot Study," *Lancet Oncology* 14, no. 11 (2013): 1112–20.

14. Elizabeth Blackburn and Elissa Epel, *The Telomere Effect* (New York: Grand Central Books, 2017).

15. Shirley Telles, Sachin Kr. Sharma, Arti Yadav, Nilkamal Singh, and Acharya Balkrishna, "A Comparative Controlled Trial Comparing the Effects of Yoga and Walking for Overweight and Obese Adults," *Medical Science Monitor* 20 (2014): 894–904.

16. Blackburn and Epel, *Telomere Effect*; Lauche et al., "A Systematic Review and Meta-analysis."

Chapter 6 Motivation, Medical Risks, Drugs, and Diets

1. Kevin D. Hall and Scott Kahan, "Maintenance of Lost Weight and Long-Term Management of Obesity," *Medical Clinics of North America* 102, no. 1 (2018): 183–97.

2. Kim E. Innes and Heather K. Vincent, "The Influence of Yoga-Based Programs on Risk Profiles in Adults with Type 2 Diabetes Mellitus: A Systematic Review," *Evidence-Based Complementary and Alternative Medicine* 4, no. 4 (2007): 469–86.

3. Maria Araneta, Matthew A. Allison, Elizabeth Barrett-Connor, and Alka M. Kanaya, "Evidence Based Diabetes Management" (paper presented at the 73rd Session of American Diabetes Association, Chicago, IL, June 21–25, 2013).

4. Ramesh Lal Bijlani, R. P. Vempati, Raj Kumar Yadav, Rooma Basu Ray, Vani Gupta, Ratna Sharma, Nalin J. Mehta, and Sushil Chandra Mahapatra, "A Brief but Comprehensive Lifestyle Education Program Based on Yoga Reduces Risk Factors for Cardiovascular Disease and Diabetes Mellitus," *Journal of Alternative and Complementary Medicine* 11, no. 2 (2005): 267–74.

5. Zu-Yao Yang, Hui-Bin Zhong, Chen Mao, Jin-Qiu Yuan, Ya-Fang Huang, Xin-Yin Wu, Yuan-Mei Gao, and Jin-Ling Tang, "Yoga for Asthma," *Cochrane Database of Systematic Reviews* 4 (April 27, 2016).

6. Bijlani et al., "A Brief but Comprehensive Lifestyle Education Program."

7. Yang et al., "Yoga for Asthma."

8. Beverly Balkau, "The DECODE Study: Diabetes Epidemiology; Collabora-

tive Analysis of Diagnostic Criteria in Europe," *Diabetes & Metabolism* 26, no. 4 (2000): 282–86.

9. Lesley Ward, Simon Stebbings, Josie Athens, Daniel Cherkin, and G. David Baxter, "Yoga for the Management of Pain and Sleep in Rheumatoid Arthritis: A Pilot Randomized Controlled Trial," *Musculoskeletal Care* 16, no. 1 (2017): 39–47.

10. Christoph Handschin and Bruce M. Spiegelman. "The Role of Exercise and PGC1α in Inflammation and Chronic Disease," *Nature* 454, no. 7203 (2008): 463–69.

11. Ward et al., "Yoga for the Management of Pain and Sleep"; Jin Lee, Hana Yoo, and Byoung-Hee Lee, "Effects of Augmented Reality–Based Otago Exercise on Balance, Gait, and Physical Factors in Elderly Women to Prevent Falls: A Randomized Controlled Trial," *Journal of Physical Therapy Science* 19, no. 9 (2017): 1586–89.

12. Christie Abagon, "Weight Loss Advice: Obese, Overweight Patients 'Less Likely to Die' after Heart Surgery," iTechPost, January 20, 2017, http://www.itechpost.com/articles/76269/20170120/weight-loss-advice -obese-overweight-patients-less-die-heart-surgery.htm; "Surgical Complications Twelve Times More Likely in Obese Patients," Johns Hopkins Medicine, June 29, 2011, https://www.hopkinsmedicine.org/news/media/ releases/surgical_complications_twelve_times_more_likely_in_obese_ patients.

13. Zia Ul-Haq, Daniel F. MacKay, Daniel Martin, Daniel J. Smith, Jason M. R. Gill, Barbara I. Nicholl, Breda Cullen, Jonathan Evans, Beverly Roberts, Ian Deary, John Gallacher, Matthew Hotopf, Nick Craddock, and Jill P. Pell, "Heaviness, Health and Happiness: A Cross-Sectional Study of 163,066 UK Biobank Participants," *Journal of Epidemiology and Community Health* 68, no. 4 (2014): 340–48.

14. Ul-Haq et al., "Heaviness, Health and Happiness."

15. See "Safety Profile," Qsymia, https://qsymia.com/hcp/safety/; and "Topiramate Side Effects," Drugs.com, https://www.drugs.com/sfx/topiramate-side -effects.html.

16. See "Suprenza," RxList, https://www.rxlist.com/suprenza-side-effects-drug -center.htm; and "Phentermine Hydrochloride—Drug Summary," Prescribers' Digital Reference, https://www.pdr.net/drug-summary/Suprenza -phentermine-hydrochloride-2413.

17. See Highlights of Prescribing Information (Saxenda), Drugs@FDA:

FDA-Approved Drugs, https://www.accessdata.fda.gov/drugsatfda_docs/label/2014/206321Orig1s000lbl.pdf.

18. See Highlights of Prescribing Information (Contrave), https://contrave.com/content/pdf/Contrave_PI.pdf (prescriber information).

19. "Xenical," RXList, https://www.rxlist.com/xenical-side-effects-drug-center.htm (professional/side effects).

20. Ul-Haq et al., "Heaviness, Health and Happiness."

21. Hall and Kahan, "Maintenance of Lost Weight and Long-Term Management of Obesity."

22. Peter Wilson, "Death of the Calorie," *Economist: 1843*, April–May 2019, https://www.1843magazine.com/features/death-of-the-calorie.

23. Amit v. Khera, Mark Chaffin, Kaitlin H. Wade, Sohail Zahid, Joseph Brancale, Rui Zia, Marina Distefano, Ozlem Senol-Cosar, Mary E. Haas, Alexander Bick, Krishna G. Aragam, Eric S. Lander, George Davey Smith, Heather Mason-Suares, Myriam Fornage, Matthew Lebo, Nicholas J. Timpson, Lee M. Kaplan, and Sekar Kathiresan, "Polygenic Prediction of Weight and Obesity Trajectories from Birth to Adulthood," *Cell* 177, no. 3 (2019): 587–96.

24. Stacy L. Haber, Omar Awwad, April Phillips, Andrew E. Park, and Tam Minh Pham, "*Garcinia cambogia* for Weight Loss," *American Journal of Health-System Pharmacy* 75, no. 2 (2018): 17–22; Giada Crescioli, Niccolò Lombardi, Alessandra Bettiol, Ettore Marconi, Filippo Risaliti, Michele Bertoni, Francesca Menniti Ippolito, Valentina Maggini, Eugenia Gallo, Fabio Firenzuoli, and Alfredo Vannacci, "Acute Liver Injury Following *Garcinia cambogia* Weight-Loss Supplementation: Case Series and Literature Review," *Internal and Emergency Medicine* 13, no. 6 (2018): 857–72.

Chapter 7 Doing the Yoga

1. For a detailed comparison of yoga's yamas and niyamas with the Ten Commandments, see Loren M. Fishman, *Trust: The Spiritual Impulse After Darwin* (Scotts Valley, CA: CreateSpace, 2014), 386–87.

2. A useful and authoritative guide to which poses are contraindicated for which medical conditions can be found at the Yoga Injury Prevention website, www.YIP.guru.

3. Loren Fishman, MD, *Healing Yoga* (New York: W. W. Norton, 2014), 57–65.

4. B.K.S. Iyengar, *Light on Yoga* (New York: Schocken Books, 1963), 155.

Chapter 8 Staying Safe to Gain the Benefits

1. Loren Fishman, Ellen Saltonstall, and Susan Genis, "Understanding and Preventing Yoga Injuries," *International Journal of Yoga Therapy* 19, no. 1 (2009): 47–53.
2. Stephen Penman, Marc Cohen, Philip Stevens, and Sue Jackson, "Yoga in Australia: Results of a National Survey," *International Journal of Yoga* 5, no. 2 (2012): 92–101.

Chapter 9 How to Design and Use Pose Sequences

1. B.K.S. Iyengar, *Light on Yoga* (New York: Schocken Books, 1963).
2. Loren M. Fishman and Ellen Saltonstall, *Yoga for Osteoporosis* (New York: W. W. Norton, 2010).
3. Yogani, *Advanced Yoga Practices: Easy Lessons for Ecstatic Living* (Nashville, TN: AYP Publishing, 2004).

Chapter 10 From the Practical to the Sublime

1. Olya Bullard and Rajesh V. Manchanda, "How Goal Progress Influences Regulatory Focus in Goal Pursuit," *Journal of Consumer Psychology* 27, no. 3 (2017): 302–17.
2. Jack London, *The Call of the Wild and White Fang*, Clydesdale Classics (New York: Simon & Schuster, 2016), Kindle edition.
3. Agence France-Presse, "Yoga Joins UNESCO World Heritage List," *Guardian*, December 1, 2016, https://www.theguardian.com/lifeandstyle/2016/dec/01/yoga-joins-unesco-intangible-world-heritage-list.
4. For a further discussion of this, see Loren M. Fishman, *Trust: The Spiritual Impulse After Darwin* (Scotts Valley, CA: CreateSpace, 2014), 386–87.